# IMPLEMENTING GP FUNDHOLDING

## STATE OF HEALTH SERIES

Edited by Chris Ham, Director of Health Services Management Centre, University of Birmingham

# IMPLEMENTING GP FUNDHOLDING
## Wild Card or Winning Hand?

**Howard Glennerster,
Manos Matsaganis and
Patricia Owens
with Stephanie Hancock**

**Open University Press**
Buckingham · Philadelphia

Open University Press
Celtic Court
22 Ballmoor
Buckingham
MK18 1XW

and
1900 Frost Road, Suite 101
Bristol, PA 19007, USA

First Published 1994

A catalogue record of this book is available from the British Library

*Library of Congress Cataloging-in-Publication Data*

Implementing GP fundholding  wild card or winning hand? / Howard
    Glennerster . . . [et al.].
        p.    cm. – (The State of health series)
    Includes bibliographical references and index.
    ISBN 0–335–19334–X    ISBN 0–335–19108–8 (pbk.)
    1. Fundholding (Medical economics)—Great Britain.
I. Glennerster, Howard. II. Series.
RA410,55.G7I47 1994
362.1′068′1—dc20                                        94–27679
                                                            CIP

Typeset by Type Study, Scarborough
Printed in Great Britain by St Edmundsbury Press
Bury St Edmunds, Suffolk

# CONTENTS

# SERIES EDITOR'S INTRODUCTION

Health services in many developed countries have come under critical scrutiny in recent years. In part this is because of increasing expenditure, much of it funded from public sources, and the pressure this has put on governments seeking to control public spending. Also important has been the perception that resources allocated to health services are not always deployed in an optimal fashion. Thus at a time when the scope for increasing expenditure is extremely limited, there is a need to search for ways of using existing budgets more efficiently. A further concern has been the desire to ensure access to health care of various groups on an equitable basis. In some countries this has been linked to a wish to enhance patient choice and to make service providers more responsive to patients as 'consumers'.

Underlying these specific concerns are a number of more fundamental developments which have a significant bearing on the performance of health services. Three are worth highlighting. First, there are demographic changes, including the ageing population and the decline in the proportion of the population of working age. These changes will both increase the demand for health care and at the same time limit the ability of health services to respond to this demand.

Second, advances in medical science will also give rise to new demands within the health services. These advances cover a range of possibilities, including innovations in surgery, drug therapy, screening and diagnosis. The pace of innovation is likely to quicken as the end of the century approaches, with significant implications for the funding and provision of services.

Third, public expectations of health services are rising as those who use services demand higher standards of care. In part, this is stimulated by developments within the health service, including the availability of new technology. More fundamentally, it stems from the emergence of a more educated and informed population, in which people are accustomed to being treated as consumers rather than patients.

Against this background, policymakers in a number of countries are reviewing the future of health services. Those countries which have traditionally relied on a market in health care are making greater use of regulation and planning. Equally, those countries which have traditionally relied on regulation and planning are moving towards a more competitive approach. In no country is there complete satisfaction with existing methods of financing and delivery, and everywhere there is a search for new policy instruments.

The aim of this series is to contribute to debate about the future of health services through an analysis of major issues in health policy. These issues have been chosen because they are both of current interest and of enduring importance. The series is intended to be accessible to students and informed lay readers as well as to specialists working in this field. The aim is to go beyond a textbook approach to health policy analysis and to encourage authors to move debate about their issue forward. In this sense, each book presents a summary of current research and thinking, and an exploration of future policy directions.

Professor Chris Ham
Director of Health Services Management Centre,
University of Birmingham

# PREFACE

The changes to the National Health Service that were initiated by Mrs Thatcher's Government in the 1989 White Paper *Working for Patients* (Department of Health, 1989a) were the most far reaching since the service began. The Government itself seemed reluctant to initiate any evaluation of the changes except in Scotland (Howie, 1992; 1993). The King's Fund decided to fill the gap and commissioned a series of research projects on different parts of the reforms (Robinson and Le Grand, 1994). Our project was to monitor the process of implementing GP fundholding, which turned out to be the most controversial part of the reforms, as well as the most radical. We chose a group of intending fundholders before the legislation was even passed and have followed their fortunes ever since, adding practices from the third wave, too. We should like to thank all these GPs, their practice managers and other staff who have been so patient, helpful and generous with their time. We have also had full and friendly co-operation from regional staff in the three regions we studied in detail and from FHSA managers, district, unit and trust staff whom we also interviewed.

Stephanie Hancock stepped in in the final year of the project and did a first rate job of interviewing and acting as research assistant. Maria Benedicta-Edwards provided most of the material on which Chapter 7 was based. It would not have been completed without her. Jane Dickson coped with our drafts and supported us with her usual quiet and cheerful competence throughout. The Suntory–Toyota International Centre for Economics and Related Disciplines at the London School of Economics provided the perfect research environment. Our spouses gave us the understanding support without which no such enterprise can succeed.

# 1

# FUNDHOLDING: A MICROCOSM OF THE FUTURE?

In part, this book is about a relatively restricted, if controversial, element in the United Kingdom's 1991 health care reforms – general practice fundholding. On another level it reflects a much wider move towards contracting and competition in health and social services not only in the United Kingdom but internationally. It also highlights the dilemmas this new form of social policy will pose.

The oil shocks of the 1970s and their aftermath checked the almost continuous growth of state welfare that had followed the second world war. For 30 years virtually all advanced economies had expanded the share of their national incomes devoted to social programmes. In the United Kingdom the share of gross domestic product (GDP) spent on social services rose from 15 per cent in 1945 to 25 per cent in 1975. Very similar, indeed stronger, trends were evident in other countries (Glennerster, 1992). One of the major components of this upward trend was health expenditure. On average, in all Organization for Economic Co-operation and Development (OECD) countries, health expenditure rose 60 per cent faster than national incomes in the period 1960 to 1975 (OECD, 1987). Most of this growth was financed from public funds, although the rates of increase were somewhat greater in countries with a large private sector.

It was the 1970s oil crises that broke this trend. Initially the changed economic climate did not produce structural change. For a decade or more governments followed a policy of belt-tightening rather than radical reform. Health expenditure was kept in check, yet the pressures that had fuelled the post-war expansion were still present. More severe rationing of health care, in one form or another, followed. The political costs that were involved led many governments to look at radical structural change in their health care systems (Hurst, 1991; OECD, 1992b; Saltman and von Otter, 1992). They wanted their varied health care systems to produce more within a restricted budget. The issues were perhaps most lucidly set out in a report by the Dutch Government Committee on Choices in Health Care (1992).

Fiscal constraint was only one force at work. Increasingly the old structures, dating back to the immediate post-war period, were beginning to show their age. Many, and especially those in the so-called 'advanced' welfare states of the United Kingdom and northern Europe, reflected a statist view of social policy that had been prevalent in the 1940s but was increasingly out of tune with the consumerism of the 1990s. The failures of market capitalism in the 1930s and the relative success of the central state in mobilizing support in the second world war in the United Kingdom further helped to shape its collective welfare institutions of the 1940s.

Universal services run by a single bureaucratic agency gave the promise of equal treatment and equal access. This was rarely achieved (Le Grand, 1982). Achieved or not, it tended to be at the cost of consumer choice, which was becoming the touchstone of a wide range of services in the private sector. That consumerism may, in the eyes of critics, seem somewhat false, but the capacity to shop around in housing, insurance, financial services and supermarkets contrasted increasingly favourably with the take it or leave it attitudes of public services.

The powerlessness of consumers, their incapacity to take their custom elsewhere – to use the sanction of 'exit' – meant that social services gradually became complacent and unresponsive (Hirschman, 1970). Power shifted to the professions who controlled the services. Structures evolved that enhanced their working conditions, not the user's satisfaction (Power, 1987). This was a gradual but insidious process. In the 1960s and 1970s attempts were made to increase users' influence through various kinds of consumer participation or through enhanced complaints procedures. Neither proved entirely satisfactory, least of all in the health services.

In the 1980s economic liberalism began to grow in appeal for just these reasons. The collapse of the command economies in Eastern Europe had a profound impact on the climate of ideas about forms of welfare. In its radical form the new economic liberalism would have abolished the state welfare institutions of the post-war period.

Yet, despite people's frustrations with these institutions, support for their original goals remained strong in many countries (Jowell *et al.*, 1989), especially in the United Kingdom, and especially about health care.

What emerged from this climate was a new paradigm, the claim that it was possible to increase consumers' satisfaction and the efficiency of these services, while keeping the principle of free and equal access. What politician could resist?

## A NEW PARADIGM?

This strategy involved keeping state finance to preserve equal access but introducing an element of competition into service provision. It has been variously labelled as the introduction of 'quasi-markets' (Le Grand *et al.*, 1991; Le Grand and Bartlett, 1993) 'market-type mechanisms' (OECD, 1992a) or 'planned markets' (Saltman and von Otter, 1992). In the United States the approach is invested with a more appealing title – 'reinventing government' (Osborne and Gaebler, 1992). Nowhere has this approach been more widely adopted than in the field of health care, where both the fiscal constraints and the deficiencies of monopolistic social agencies had become most evident (OECD, 1992b).

The extent of the competitive dose has, however, varied. One version confines the competition to suppliers of services. A public authority purchases services on behalf of all its population. Monopoly remains on the demand side. Consumers, as individuals, have no greater choice. They may gain cheaper or better services but only if the purchaser fully reflects their preferences.

A second version takes the competitive logic further. Individuals ought to be able to *choose* which purchaser they will patronize. It is only this more extreme model that fully meets the urge to make the consumer king that motivated many reformers. It is the model of the Health Maintenance Organization (HMO) in the United States where members join, pay a premium and the HMO buys hospital and other care for them. We find examples of both kinds of competition in Western health care reforms – supply-side only and supply- and demand-side competition.

In a previous volume in this series, Saltman and von Otter (1992) chart the way public health care systems in Scandinavia, eastern Europe and the United Kingdom had moved in similar directions, introducing an element of competition between public providers. Local agencies of the state retained the duty of ensuring that their populations had universal access to health care and they chose between competing hospitals or other public providers to supply services for these populations. The county councils in Sweden and the municipalities in Finland are beginning to do this. Saltman and von Otter (1992) argue that the combination of needs-based purchasing power with decentralized consumer choice enhances the modern polity, creating what they call a 'civil democracy'.

In the Netherlands the aim is to combine universal access with the right of the Dutch citizen to choose between alternative health insurance agencies (Dutch Ministry of Welfare, Health and Cultural Affairs, 1988). Similar ideas lie behind President Clinton's reform package (White House Domestic Policy Council, 1993).

The British reforms, as we shall see in more detail in Chapter 2, unusually embody elements of both these alternative models of competition. District health authorities purchase on behalf of their whole populations – their populations have no choice about what they receive. GP fundholding gives patients the choice of purchaser. The British debate on the NHS is, therefore, just part of a much wider international discussion on the very future of social policy. The changes to the NHS, like other reforms in Sweden and Finland, challenge the old command and control paradigm of social welfare. They decentralize purchasing power without going the whole way to a private consumer market. Yet, as we shall see, consumer choice and competition carry dangers as well as advantages. There are difficult trade-offs to be made between improving efficiency and ensuring fairness, between the capacity to plan and the scope for innovation. GP fundholding encapsulates, in one experiment, many of the dilemmas of the new social policy paradigm evolving not just in the United Kingdom but in many other countries too (Taylor-Gooby and Lawson, 1993).

## THE FUTURE OF PRIMARY CARE

If the future of social policy is one underlying theme in this story, the future of primary health care is another. The local family doctor is an unusual but critically important feature of the British health service. He or she acts as the gatekeeper to the whole of the rest of the elaborate specialist services. Ninety per cent of all health care episodes begin and end with the individual's own GP. Where the GP is a good one this personal service is a much valued part of the NHS and one the Swedes, for example, despite their strong primary health care system, are thinking of copying (Glennerster and Matsaganis, 1992). A British citizen cannot gain access to an NHS hospital except with a letter of referral from his or her GP, excluding an accident or emergency. In many other health care systems the public has direct access to expensive specialists. This GP gatekeeping function is one of the reasons why the British health system is relatively cost effective and personal.

Yet, at the same time, general practice has many deficiencies. In the course of this research the authors have visited practices in a wide variety of settings. If we had been visitors from Mars we should have found it inconceivable that they were all part of a single national service. The harassed practice in a deprived area with rude and angry receptionists, a crowded and sullen waiting room with a drunk on the doorstep, contrasted with large, well-run rural and suburban practices where calm good humour prevailed, children played in the toddlers' corner, rose beds bloomed in the drive and branch clinics were linked by computer. And all that before fundholding!

Although it was Aneurin Bevan's intention that the NHS should have a powerful primary health care foundation, general practice has remained a weak partner in the British health care system, isolated from the other community health services, which were first run by local authorities and then, after 1974, by separate bureaucracies within the district health authority. This separation makes talk of a 'Primary Health Care Team' of community nurses, health visitors, other professionals and GPs, a fiction. Good working relations developed in many practices, despite these organizational barriers but, as we have found, many GPs do not even know what their non-medical colleagues are doing or which of their patients were being seen by whom.

Over a long period GPs lost power and status to the growing dominance of the hospital and the hospital consultant. This was not just a reflection of changes in medicine, the coming of the NHS itself had hastened the change. The consultants in the old voluntary, fee-paying hospitals depended for their income on patients referred by the GP. In the new NHS the consultant was paid a salary and had the power to pick and choose the patients to take from a long waiting list. The GP became a supplicant pleading with the consultant on behalf of his or her patient. Professor Richard Titmuss of the

London School of Economics (LSE) used to joke in his lectures that one of the important consequences of the coming of the NHS in 1948 was that prior to that time consultants sent Christmas cards to GPs but after that the opposite happened. This sense of professional status rivalry runs through this story too.

In the 1980s medical technology began to change direction. Massive invasive surgery began to be replaced by techniques that could be done in local hospitals, even in day wards. Outpatient diagnostic work could be done outside the hospital as small-scale and cheap equipment could be installed in local surgeries. The Chinese walls between hospital and primary health care began to crumble. Yet, so long as quite separate budgets remained firmly allocated to hospitals, to community services, to GPs and to social services departments, there was little incentive to question the logic of these walls.

GP fundholding was to open up this possibility.

Thus, we have to see the fundholding experiment against this backdrop of pressure for greater consumerism and change in health care technology. These factors are at work not just in the United Kingdom but world wide. That is why it has aroused such interest abroad (Swedish Committee on the Funding and Organization of Health Services and Medical Care, 1993).

Information technology gave small-scale organizations the capacity to manage large budgets, to individualize the billing of diverse providers, to track their patient population and its movement between primary and secondary and more specialist care. This had been pioneered by Health Maintenance Organizations (HMOs) in the United States.

Other predisposing factors were at work. The UK Treasury was worried about primary care for quite different reasons. It had managed to put cash limits or global budget ceilings on hospital and community health services in the 1970s but it had never succeeded in doing so for primary care. This was a demand-led service. It was not possible to stop patients going to their GP. How could you stop GPs prescribing drugs for their patients? The result was that the primary health care budget in the 1980s expanded faster than any other part of the NHS budget, and the pharmaceutical part of this budget expanded the fastest of all. The Treasury was interested in trying to cash-limit that growth. These concerns also lay behind the Government's determination to impose a contract on GPs (Day, 1992).

## THE ORIGINS OF THE FUNDHOLDING IDEA

The idea of giving general practitioners the capacity to buy hospital services on behalf of their patients predated the Conservative Government's White Paper on the reform of the NHS (Department of Health, 1989a).

The principle had been discussed by Alan Maynard, Professor of Health Economics at York University, in the early 1980s, and was presented to a seminar organized by the Office of Health Economics (Maynard, 1986). Maynard had always been an advocate of market solutions in health and education but he recognized, like most other health economists, that there were features of health markets that did not fit the assumptions needed for a free market to work efficiently (Barr *et al.*, 1988). Not least of the problems was the fact that patients lacked the knowledge to be informed purchasers of health care. They were reliant on professional advisers to tell them whether they needed a service and from whom to get it. In the NHS, GPs were those advisers. Why not give them the task of buying services on their patients' behalf? This would combine consumer choice and competition between GPs and hospitals for the patients' custom. The idea drew upon the American HMO model we have mentioned before, which was very much in favour with Washington policymakers in the early 1980s (Brown, 1983). Viewed from the American standpoint it restricted patients' total freedom of choice to go to any specialist of their choice directly, but compared to the NHS it put much more power in the hands of the consumer.

There had been diverse origins to this movement in the United States. Some began as worker-owned health co-operatives that pooled members' resources to ensure some health care even in times of low earnings. The lumber workers of the American North West were one example; industrial workers of the mid-West did the same. Then employers who needed a healthy labour force organized something on similar lines. The now huge Kaiser Permanente scheme began with workers employed on the Federal dam construction projects of the 1930s.

The essence of the HMO approach is that members pay a fixed annual premium to a group of doctors who pool this revenue and aim to provide a comprehensive range of medical care for their members. To do this they may buy in services on a contract basis from local private or non-profit hospitals, or do the work themselves. What attracted the notice of economists was that the pre-paid premium basis of funding set a ceiling to what could be spent in any one year and gave the doctors an incentive to keep costs down and to promote good health and conservative medicine. Two members of the Department of Health (DoH) who visited the United States at this time were struck by the freedom this form of funding gave to GPs and the leverage it gave them over hospitals. They returned home keen to see how these principles might be applied to British general practice. (For an account of the differences between fundholding and HMOs see Weiner and Ferriss, 1990.)

Prompted partly by the Treasury's concerns, the Government had instituted a review of primary care in the mid-1980s. This produced a Green Paper for discussion and then the White Paper *Promoting Better Health* (Department of Health and Social Services, 1987). It was this that led to the enforced contract for GPs in 1990. In the early discussions in 1984 Mrs Thatcher's No. 10 Policy Unit picked up Alan Maynard's idea and pursued it while the DHSS developed its thoughts on HMOs. The result was the very first version of the fundholding idea. This found its way into the draft Green Paper but was left out at the last moment as too radical. Nevertheless, the junior health minister at the time, Kenneth Clarke, must have been aware of it.

This was not the only or the most important force for reform, however. The NHS seemed to many in the Conservative Party the last bastion of a socialist past and the most difficult to shift. An American economist who had been a powerful advocate of competitive reforms to heath care in the United States was invited to visit and comment on the NHS. He criticized its unresponsive and inflexible tendencies while praising its capacity to provide universal access (Enthoven, 1985). He advocated a version of the reforms he had been advocating at home – district health authorities would become large HMOs purchasing health care from whatever hospitals could provide a good service at a competitive price.

When Mrs Thatcher set up the National Health Service Review in 1987 this Enthoven model became the front runner for change (for an account of the origins of the reforms, and the discussions on them, see Butler, 1992). Some right-wing think tanks suggested more radical options – giving tax relief to private health insurance, going over to a private insurance model altogether (Letwyn and Redwood, 1988; Pirie and Butler, 1988). These were discussed by the review team but eliminated fairly early on according to Mrs Thatcher in her memoirs (Thatcher, 1993). Most middle-range experts advocated some version of the district-based purchasing model (Robinson, 1988). The case for smaller GP-based HMOs was advocated by David Willetts and Michael Goldsmith (1988) in a pamphlet for the Centre for Policy Studies.

By the summer of 1988 Mrs Thatcher's Policy Unit was worried that the discussions were becoming bogged down and the proposals on the table less and less radical. They reintroduced the old GP funding idea (Thatcher, 1993). It was at this point that Mrs Thatcher replaced John Moore as Secretary of State for Health with Kenneth Clarke. The old GP purchasing scheme was taken down and dusted off. It then became very much Mr Clarke's own initiative but its late arrival in the discussions explains why it was never fully integrated into the whole and why it was so rudimentary in outline, having the appearance of an appendage to the basic reform package in which the districts emerged as the main actors. That is certainly the way most regional officers saw the 'GP experiment' in 1990 when we first interviewed them.

## ADAPTING THE HMO IDEA TO THE UNITED KINGDOM

Transposing the HMO model to the United Kingdom posed real difficulties. There was simply no comparably large primary care organization. Most HMOs in the United States are very large by the standard of British general practice; many are as large as a district health authority, some larger. American experience suggested that small HMOs were financially vulnerable. An unfortunately large number of expensive patients needing emergency treatment in any one year could bankrupt a small HMO. To average out this possibility the 'risk pool' needs to be large. The American work suggested that HMOs were at risk if their patient list was less than 50,000 or so (Weiner and Ferriss, 1990). No British practice came anywhere near that size; only about 40 per cent of practices had more than 7000 patients.

Other research in the United States suggested that the flat rate premium produced other problems. Some patients cost a lot more than others and could be predicted to cost more. For that reason doctors were reluctant to take them on to their books – a process called biased selection or cream skimming (Luft and Miller, 1988).

Those in the DoH working on the reforms were well aware of

these problems and attempted to build into the scheme a set of safeguards. First, the scheme was to be confined to large practices. The White Paper (Department of Health, 1989a, p. 49) said the scheme would apply to practices with 'at least 11,000 patients'. This limit was lowered to 9000 in 1990 and to 7000 in 1992.

Second, the budget was only to cover non-emergency care. Most of the treatments the GP could buy from the hospital were to cover standard, relatively inexpensive procedures, and excluded any open-ended treatment that might result from a GP's referral for a simple case. The White Paper said the range of services GPs could buy would include all outpatient care, diagnostic tests and a restricted range of inpatient and day case treatments 'such as hip replacements and cataract removals, for which there may be some choice over time and place of treatment'. It was not until much later that the DoH worked out a full list of treatments covered by the scheme (see Appendix 1).

It is important to emphasize this restricted scope because it gives rise to much misunderstanding. It meant that only about 15 per cent of the total cost of hospital care would pass through fundholders' hands even assuming all GPs became fundholders. In 1992 only 2 per cent of hospitals' budgets were being bought by fundholding GPs.

Finally, the scheme included what insurers would call a 'stop loss' provision. Notwithstanding the relative cheapness of the treatments covered, if a single patient were to cost the practice more than £5000 the extra cost would be met by the district health authority.

There were, in short, major safeguards designed to avoid the kinds of financial disasters that had hit small HMOs in the United States. The scheme is described in more detail in Chapter 2.

## WHAT WERE THE OBJECTIVES OF THE REFORM?

It is clear that the scheme that emerged in the White Paper had been watered down considerably from the original Maynard plan, which would have had GPs buy all the hospital and other services their patients needed from a budget given out by central government. Maynard's scheme would have covered every GP; fundholding was to cover only some GPs and their patients. However, the scheme *was* targeted on those parts of the NHS that had produced the greatest criticism. Many of those involved saw it as a kind of vanguard efficiency device.

● *Non-emergency treatment.* NHS patients who face life-threatening conditions or need emergency treatment get it fairly rapidly. What the NHS has been very bad at is treating non-emergency but painful or hampering conditions – the hip replacements and cataract operations mentioned by the White Paper. In these cases treatment is repetitive, if the hospital team did more operations under the old pattern of finance they merely worked harder and suffered more stress; there was no real incentive to do more. On the contrary if a consultant had a private clinic there was a strong incentive not to treat patients too speedily but to keep a long waiting list and encourage those who could afford it to get quicker treatment privately. As we shall see, many of our GPs thought this was a major reason why some clinicians' waiting times were so long and why it was these consultants who were most angry about their becoming fundholders. Thus the fact that GPs were allowed to buy only a restricted range of procedures did not mean they were insignificant. If the GPs did succeed in improving matters, they would be the key to removing much of the popular criticism and inequity in the service which derive from precisely this range of treatments.

● *Outpatients.* Once again this is a poor relation in the NHS. The outpatient clinic comes low on most hospital consultants' order of priorities. Appointments schemes are poorly run, waiting times are long and large numbers of patients do not turn up. Yet, after the GP, outpatient clinics are the most frequent contact patients have with the service. If they could be improved it would go a long way to improving the image of the NHS and overall patient satisfaction.

● *Drugs budgets.* For different reasons this was also a priority to government. The rising costs of this element have been discussed already. It was felt that if GPs were given more budget freedom overall they might be prepared to accept a cash limit on their drugs spending and hence meet the Treasury's economy objective.

● *Referrals.* Some in government were also concerned about the wide disparity in GP referral patterns. Some GPs referred far fewer patients to hospital than others for reasons that were difficult to explain. Hospitals were, to GPs, 'free goods'. If GPs had to consider the costs of their referrals they might refer fewer patients.

The origins of the scheme were, therefore, varied and somewhat fortuitous but they did focus on some key deficiencies in the NHS. They also went farthest towards the notion of opening up the service to competition and transferring purchasing power from state bureaucracies nearer to the patient. Like all reforms the original objectives of the scheme developed as GPs themselves began to set the agenda once they had acquired their own budgets.

# 2

# THE SCHEME

## THE ORIGINAL SCHEME

The elements of the scheme finally introduced in 1991 were:

- Practices with more than 9000 patients could apply for fundholding status. Regions drew up a list of criteria to screen applicants. The aim was to ensure that they were managerially and technically capable of handling the scheme and were fully committed to it.
- Practices received a budget allocation that could only be spent on a defined set of purposes. It could not, in theory, be used to increase the doctors' income or to benefit the practice generally. This budget was not paid as cash to the practices but held by the Family Health Service Authorities (FHSAs) and released to pay hospitals when authorized by a practice. The drugs prescribed by the doctors were not paid for directly out of any cash the doctors held but were set against the cash limit fixed for the practice. Any savings under that limit could, however, be turned into an enhanced budget allocation for other elements in the budget. The intention was to put a *cordon sanitaire* around the fundholding budget, to keep it separate from the wider income-earning activities of the partnership.
- The budget allocated to the practices to buy hospital services was deducted from the allocations the district health authority would otherwise have received.

The budget consisted of five main component parts from April 1991 to March 1993:

1 *Hospital inpatient care for a restricted range of operations.* These

covered ophthalmology; ear, nose and throat; thoracic surgery; operations on the cardiovascular system; general surgery; gynaecology; orthopaedics. Details of the treatments included are listed in Appendix 1. Emergency referrals in the above categories were excluded. Budgets were set in a way that enabled the practices to purchase historic levels of service. We discuss the budget setting process in later chapters.

2 *All outpatient visits.* These were defined as 'a patient attending a hospital or clinic other than as an inpatient' or a home visit arranged by the GP. Excluded were first appointments made where treatment followed a period as an inpatient but not in the fundholding list of treatments. Chemotherapy and radiotherapy for, for example, cancer, renal dialysis and genitourinary clinics, were excluded. As for inpatient care the budget was set on the basis of an estimate of the practices' past use of these services.

3 *Diagnostic tests done on an outpatient basis.* These included blood tests, urine tests and X-rays. Breast screening under the call and recall scheme was excluded. Budgets were set on the basis of evidence collected in the previous year about the level of activity practices demanded from hospitals. The number of different types of test requested in previous years were multiplied by their expected price.

4 *Pharmaceuticals prescribed by the practice.* The drugs budget was calculated in exactly the same way as the indicative budget within which non-fundholding practices were expected to keep.

5 *Practice staff.* Again fundholders were paid the same as other GPs for their practice staff but instead of having to get approval for each staff member, and new approval each time a receptionist left, fundholders are simply given a sum of money to cover staff costs. This is added to their total budget. It gives them flexibility to save money on staff and add savings to other elements in their budget or to make savings elsewhere and employ more staff.

Though calculated separately all these budget elements were pooled. A saving on any one of them could be used to spend more under another heading.

In addition the region pays practices a management allowance to cover the cost of additional management expertise needed (£34,000 in 1993–4). Half this figure is available in the preparatory year to up-grade management and computing. The management allowance could be used to pay for the time of a practice manager or for a

part-time adviser or contract manager. It also covered the costs of
entering into the computer the financial and referral data needed to
bill hospitals and keep track of the accounts. Claims had to be made
for these items up to the specified ceiling.

A computerized accounting system was specified by the DoH,
and various private companies, after some delay, produced software for it. All referrals had to be entered so that practices could tell
what cumulative bills were being run up as well as knowing what
bills they had actually paid. It produced several kinds of monthly
and end-of-year statements, which had to be sent to the FHSA.

## 1993 EXTENSION

Early in 1992, as part of the run-up to the general election, William
Waldegrave, then the Secretary of State for Health, announced that
the scheme would be extended to include practices with only 7000
patients. This reduced size limit operated for practices joining the
scheme from April 1993, the third wave of fundholders. Two
practices with 3500 patients each could combine for fundholding
purposes. One of our third-wave practices was in this position.

From April 1993 the scope of the fund was also extended. When
explaining the changes the DoH said:

> The purpose of including these services in the fundholding
> scheme is to apply the benefits that have been derived in the
> acute sector in the first year to a wider range of services. It is
> anticipated that these benefits will include improved communi-
> cations between the professional groups; the definition of
> shared goals and objectives; a better understanding of the
> respective contributions to patient care of GPs, practice
> nurses, district nurses, health visitors and all community
> mental health workers . . . It will enable the Primary Health
> Care Team to plan more effectively for patients/clients – for
> example by transferring resources from other elements of the
> practice fund to purchase more district nursing to support early
> discharge (EL(92)261 para. 2.2).

The budget was thus extended to include, in addition to the above:
community health services; district nursing; health visiting; chiropody; dietetics; all community and outpatient mental health
services; mental health counselling; health services for people with

learning disabilities and all referrals made by health visitors, district nurses and community mental handicap nurses. Terminal care and midwifery were excluded. The health visiting and district nursing budget covered services provided for patients of the practice as well as referrals to other services made by these staff and the costs of equipment.

Budgets were to be set by regions assuming the existing levels of service plus any planned changes such as a substantial increase in the list size. Each practice would be funded for the existing level and grade of staff allocated to it. Practices would not be charged for the public health duties performed by health visitors. When calculating the prices to be charged to practices community units must include the costs of management and specialist support and training.

The DoH ruled that practices could only purchase from established NHS community units. GPs would not be allowed to employ community staff directly or through the private sector. This usually limited practices to their existing unit, except where they were on the border of two community units or trusts. There was an example of a GP using a more distant community unit.

To ease the initial problems, the form of the contract was also limited. GPs could only use fixed-price non-attributable contracts. These would not be sensitive to volume or activity levels and would not identify the costs of individual patients. It was hoped to relax some of these restrictions as information improved. Even so, many GPs complained that giving them a budget in these circumstances was merely a fiction. Their freedom was nothing like as great as with hospital services. We discuss this later.

The feeling of not being trusted was strengthened by the DoH requiring practices to gain prior approval from regions before setting contracts with community services, to ensure they were only buying from NHS units or trusts and that they were purchasing as much as last year. Neither condition applied to community psychiatric nursing or mental handicap nursing.

## PRIVATE COMPANIES

Early in the history of the scheme the DoH was faced with deciding what to do about treatments on this list that could be undertaken by GPs themselves. The DoH took the view that GPs could not pay themselves to do minor surgery beyond that already paid for within the existing regulations. They were purchasers; they must purchase from a separate entity.

Fundholders thought this unreasonable, because they claimed they could do some minor work both more cheaply and more conveniently for their patients on the premises. Some had small but well-equipped facilities for minor surgery. Several practices responded to the DoH's ban by setting up private companies, which they owned; they then argued they were separate providers. The DoH initially permitted this with controls and safeguards on price and range of procedure. Although only 50 of the 600 first- and second-wave practices set up private companies (*Fundholding*, April 7, 1993), the idea that the GPs could profit from the use of the fund provoked a lot of critical comment. In 1993 the DoH revised the rules (*GP Fundholding Practices: The Provision of Secondary Care*, HSG(93)14); private companies were to go. Instead a rather restricted list of 17 procedures was drawn up for which GPs could be paid directly from the fund in addition to those any GP could do under existing arrangements. Each partner could spend only 30 hours per month doing such work. Regions must approve such arrangements and they require fairly stringent quality and accounting standards.

## THE SCHEME'S GROWTH

In the first year of the scheme 7 per cent of the population were covered by GPs who joined the scheme. This amounted to 291 practices and 1713 actual GPs. In the second year the scope of the scheme nearly doubled covering 13 per cent of the population. In 1993, after the third wave joined, 25 per cent of the population were patients of fundholders. The total number of fundholders reached 1244 and the number of individual GPs 6057. The total budget allocated to them was £1800 million.

The population covered differed from region to region (Table 2.1). Within regions, the spread of fundholding was even more varied. In one county we studied nearly two-thirds of the population would be covered in 1994. In other areas a fundholder was rare.

In 1992–3 only about 2 per cent of the hospital budget was purchased through the agency of GPs. Even if all GPs in an area had been fundholders between 1991 and 1993 the percentage of the hospital and community service budget controlled by them would

**Table 2.1** 1993–4 GP fundholders: numbers at April 1 1993

| Region | Number of funds[1] | Number of practices | Number of groups | Number of GPs | Population covered (000s) | Percentage of the population covered |
|---|---|---|---|---|---|---|
| Northern | 69 | 72 | 3 | 392 | 763 | 25 |
| Yorkshire | 108 | 118 | 5 | 587 | 1202 | 33 |
| Trent | 138 | 159 | 11 | 736 | 1494 | 31 |
| East Anglia | 48 | 51 | 2 | 278 | 530 | 25 |
| NW Thames | 88 | 95 | 4 | 458 | 930 | 27 |
| NE Thames | 48 | 52 | 1 | 229 | 522 | 14 |
| SE Thames | 77 | 88 | 5 | 374 | 819 | 22 |
| SW Thames | 66 | 69 | 3 | 360 | 730 | 25 |
| Wessex | 54 | 57 | 3 | 325 | 645 | 22 |
| Oxford | 74 | 76 | 1 | 431 | 866 | 33 |
| South Western | 69 | 75 | 2 | 414 | 657 | 19 |
| West Midlands | 131 | 139 | 8 | 767 | 1378 | 26 |
| Mersey | 84 | 101 | 12 | 423 | 838 | 35 |
| North Western | 66 | 83 | 9 | 329 | 691 | 17 |
| England | 1120 | 1235 | 69 | 6103 | 12065 | 25 |

*Source:* returns from regions.
1. Some practices hold joint funds.

**Table 2.2** Allocations to fundholders

|  | Percentage of budget |
| --- | --- |
| Hospital and community services purchases | 49 |
| Drugs | 39 |
| Staff | 7 |
| Management allowances | 3 |
| Computing allowances | 2 |
| Total | 100 |

only have been about 15 per cent. After 1993 this potential figure rose to 20 per cent with the inclusion of community services.

Appendix 1 sets out in detail all the procedures covered by the scheme, the other elements in the budget, the rules and the Government regulations that covered the scheme in September 1993. The allocations to fundholders were made up as shown in Table 2.2.

The scheme had therefore grown rapidly in its first three years, which were covered by this study. It also looked set to grow further so long as the Conservative Government remained in power. Fourth- and potential fifth-wave applicants were numerous and the scheme was well on its way to covering half the population. However, the Labour Party was still committed to abolishing the scheme at the time of writing in 1994. It remained the most controversial part of the National Health Service Reforms.

# 3

# THE STUDY

## IMPLEMENTING A NOVEL IDEA – COULD IT WORK?

The research had two main objectives. The first was designed to be an implementation study, an account of the administrative process by which this major break with existing arrangements was carried through and an evaluation of its success in its own terms. Early in 1990 we met considerable misgivings about whether the scheme was actually feasible. Others in the service argued that it should only be tried as a limited experiment, so novel was it. Could it be carried through? What would have to be adapted or abandoned?

The political scientists have changed their simplified models of how public policies are implemented. The early work followed an engineering analogy. Central or Federal Government set out a blue print, which lower agencies followed rather as a builder follows an architect's drawings. Success could be measured in terms of the extent to which the original specifications were followed. Later writers challenged this view. Elmore (1978, 1982) argued that original intentions of central agencies were often modified, especially where a great deal of discretion lay with the service providers (Lipsky, 1980). Their knowledge of the practical constraints was usually more detailed than the legislators' or the central bureaucrats'. Judging success in top-down terms could therefore be misleading. Adaptation to revealed difficulties would be more realistic (Hill, 1993). This was the spirit in which we approached the first objective of the study.

## WHICH THEORY OF CONTRACTING WOULD FIT BEST?

The second element in the research took economics, not political science, as its starting point. As we saw in Chapter 1, the health reforms in the United Kingdom derived from two competing paradigms of how best to structure the market for health. Both rejected the proposition that individuals should simply be left to purchase their own health care through third party health insurance. Both argued that the purchasing and providing functions should be split. Where they differed was in who should do the purchasing. There were arguments of efficiency and equity involved.

### Efficiency arguments

The economic efficiency advantages claimed for district purchasing by Enthoven (1985) and many of those we interviewed were:

- Districts would be able to look comprehensively at the needs of their areas and make consistent rational priorities on the basis of maximizing health gains to the population in the area at minimum cost. GPs were not in a position to look at the needs of the whole area.
- Districts would be able to judge which providers were able to give the best and most cost-effective care. As they had the expertise it would be administratively cheaper for all the contracting to be done by one agency. Separate contracting by small practices would be administratively costly.
- Where some major changes were necessary in the pattern of service delivery, districts would be in the best position to manage the change – the run-down of a local hospital, for example.
- Districts would be large purchasers and able to act as monopsonist, powerful purchasers in their own areas; GPs would be weak purchasers.
- If GPs' budgets were set on a per capita basis like HMOs, fundholding GPs would have an incentive to 'cream skim' or avoid taking the most expensive patients.
- The practices were too small. The claims on their budgets would fluctuate from one year to the next. There would be many surpluses on the one hand and overspends on the other; practices would go bankrupt.

● Fundholders would also have an incentive to under-refer their patients to hospital and make profits at their patients' expense.

In contrast, Maynard's efficiency case for GP-based purchasing was based on a different set of economic theories, which drew, implicitly at least, on public choice theory. It was outlined in a seminar to the Welfare State Programme at the LSE in November 1988. We elaborate on it here in our own language!

The district-based model still relied on a centralized rational planning approach. It assumed that districts had good information to make priority decisions and would act as rational agents. The economics of contracting and of bureaucracies suggested this was far from true. As Carol Propper (1993) was to put it later:

> The central problem is the asymmetry of information between provider and purchaser under a contracting relationship. The separation of purchaser and provider means that the purchaser has less information about the technology and conditions of production than the provider. The provider can exploit this to extract rent from the purchaser and/or engage in inefficient production, so increasing the amount the purchaser has to pay for a given level of the service.

The information districts had would always be poor relative to the hospital consultants. Moreover, they were under no pressure to improve their information or their contracting because their populations were captive, unless they decided to move house. GPs as purchasers had certain advantages:

● They had better information about patients' preferences, they saw patients daily, in contrast to planners in district offices. They heard patients' complaints and experiences. They had to look after patients after discharge and learned at first hand about their experiences and could see the medical consequences. They got to know where the best consultants were.
● Moreover, GPs themselves suffered from slow or inefficient care given to their patients by a hospital. The patient landed back in the GP's surgery, taking time and resources. GPs therefore had the personal motivation to seek more efficient hospital services; district officers did not. District planners were driven by epidemiology and population figures, which was all they had and all they were trained to use.

- GPs had a self-interest in getting patients treated quickly. Frustrated and complaining patients who were waiting in pain for treatment were a drain on the GPs' time and nervous energy. Such pressure was not felt by the district planner.
- GPs could take marginal decisions to buy or not buy services from a hospital or community trust. These would give signals to the providers and the districts about changing patterns of demand and dissatisfaction with quality. GPs would not have inhibitions about using their power of exit. Districts, on the other hand, would find it politically difficult to cancel big contracts to local hospitals. It would be easier to continue close ties with existing providers with whom district officers had close historical links. The status quo would be less work and less dangerous politically.
- Above all, GPs faced competition from other GPs for their custom, limited perhaps but real at the margin in many areas. Thus patients who did not like their GP's contracts with hospitals could go to another GP. The theory of free markets depends on there being a multiplicity of both purchasers and providers (Le Grand and Bartlett, 1993). This gives the chance of diversity, innovation and competition in purchasing. Without it districts could simply lapse into monopolist tendencies.
- The combination of the hospital budget with the primary care budget gave the opportunity for trade-offs to be made between the two. The same could be said of the boundary line between community services and GPs. While each had a separate budget, organizational self-interest and traditional budget politics would prevent change.
- The inclusion of drugs spending within the budget gave a real incentive for GPs to think about their spending levels and whether to spend less on drugs and more on therapy, for example. While drugs appeared free to the GP, there was no such incentive to think holistically or economically about their use.
- The same argument applied to the cost of hospital care. Those who had advocated HMOs in the United States had argued that an annual budget ceiling made doctors think seriously about their use of hospital services and gave them an incentive to promote the health of their patients.

**Equity arguments**

From the outset the gravest criticisms of fundholding concerned its impact on the equitable distribution of health resources. Critics argued:

● The creation of two kinds of general practitioner financed in different ways would divide the health service.
● The fundholding GPs would be favoured with extra resources in order to attract them into the scheme.
● Fundholders would be able to demand preferential treatment, better and quicker, from the hospitals. This would create a two-tier service.
● Only the best-organized practices would be able to enter the scheme. If there were advantages they would only be available to patients of already well-run practices.
● Above all, the critics argued that the capitation-based funding and competition between practices would lead to GPs turning away more costly patients.
● It would also lead them to under-treat costly patients.

Fundholding enthusiasts argued that all practices should become fundholders and that competitive pressures would bring more equity than any regulations under the old system.

There were, therefore, fundamental differences of view about how the scheme would come to work in practice grounded in different economic and political views of the world.


## THE RESEARCH

The research, funded by the King's Fund as part of a programme of work on the NHS reforms, was designed to test these theories, hopes and fears. It was, essentially, a study of administrative process and the working of local health markets, not of health outcomes. That would have required a far larger research budget and a different disciplinary starting point. Would the market work in the way its advocates predicted? Would fundholders prove better contractors than districts? Would they manage to keep within budget? Would their prescribing patterns change? How would fundholding affect the internal practice organization and approach to care? Was there any evidence of cream skimming?

The study concentrated on three regions, two in London and the home counties and one predominantly rural. One region had within it the highest concentration of fundholding GPs in one FHSA anywhere in the country. We interviewed those administering the scheme in other regions but most closely followed events in these three.

Region A had 13 first-wave fundholders, 10 second-wavers and 29 third-wavers. Region B had 23 first-wavers, 21 second-wavers and 45 third-wavers. Region C, the rural region, had 9 first-wavers, 4 second-wavers and 41 third-wavers.

We chose a sample of 17 practices that had expressed interest in joining the scheme early in 1990 and reflected the range of different kinds of practice and geographical spread. Our research officer accompanied the regional officers on initial visits to intending practices. Two felt, in the end, they did not want to collaborate with the research because of the time they thought it would take. We continued to interview five, but they decided against joining the first wave. We also interviewed other practices opposed to the whole idea of fundholding. This left us with ten practices that became first-wave fundholders and that have continued in the scheme to the time when this account was completed – September 1993.

In 1991 we were asked to study a small, 8000-patient, second-wave practice that was part of the national experiment with small practices. We studied this practice intensively in its preparatory and post-fundholding year and a half.

In 1992 we chose another sample of 16 practices from those expressing an intention to join the third wave in April 1993; all did become third-wavers. We interviewed them at regular intervals in the period before and after becoming fundholders. We again interviewed a comparison group of non-fundholders.

Table 3.1 gives a brief outline of the fundholding sample practices' characteristics.

We interviewed those in the DoH responsible for the scheme, regional officers in the three regions, FHSA officials, one or more of the GP partners and the practice manager in the sample practices every three months for the first 18 months and then reduced the frequency later in the project to once every six months. We used a semi-structured one and a half to two hour interview. We attended meetings of fundholding groups and meetings of fundholders with regional officers setting the budgets. We were able to attend all the planning meetings that determined the detailed implementation of the scheme in one region. We attended seminars, workshops and conferences to make sure our emerging ideas were not inconsistent with views expressed by GPs in the rest of the country. We collected

**Table 3.1**    Sample practices' characteristics

| Practice | Partners | Locations | Patients |
|----------|----------|-----------|----------|
| *First wave* | | | |
| 1 | 3 | Inner London (not poor) | 9500 |
| 2 | 6 | Small town | 16000 |
| 3 | 5 | Large town (deprived) | 12800 |
| 4 | 6 | Large town | 12500 |
| 5 | 5 | Village/rural | 9100 |
| 6 | 6 | Small town | 13500 |
| 7 | 6 | Village/rural | 13500 |
| 8 | 6 | Village/rural | 11000 |
| 9 | 6 | Outer London (mixed ethnic/poor) | 15200 |
| 10 | 4 | Outer London | 10500 |
| *Second wave* | | | |
| 1 | 4 | Inner London (not poor) | 8000 |
| *Third Wave* | | | |
| 1 | 5 | Inner London | 10000 |
| 2 | 2 | Outer London suburbs | 3200 |
| 3 | 4 | Inner London (not poor) | 9000 |
| 4 | 6 | Small town | 11000 |
| 5 | 3 | Small town | 7000 |
| 6 | 3 | Large town | 7800 |
| 7 | 6 | Village/rural | 11000 |
| 8 | 6 | Outer London (poor) | 12500 |
| 9 | 4 | Outer London | 7400 |
| 10 | 4 | Outer London (poor) | 7500 |
| 11 | 7 | Large town (poor) | 12230 |
| 12 | 3 | Village/rural | 6500 |
| 13 | 6 | City | 13000 |
| 14 | 6 | Small town (semi-rural) | 11500 |
| 15 | 8 | Town | 13500 |
| 16 | 6 | Town | 7500 |

all the summary financial and PACT (i.e. prescription analysis and cost) data from our practices on a monthly basis and a range of documentary and statistical material about them. Regions and FHSAs were also helpful with aggregate data. This enabled us to track how well the practices were keeping to their target budgets.

We collected details of the contracts made by the practices in each year and discussed the process of negotiating the contracts with them in depth. We interviewed the providers in several of the areas, too, to see how they felt about fundholders' separate contracting powers. How had it affected their service? We followed one particular practice – a small one – in particular depth, seeing them about every two weeks.

Finally, in order to throw more light on the expense of particular patients, we enlisted the support of one of our practices. We drew a one in ten sample of their practice population, randomly drawn from the patient list. They summarized all the medical history and screening information they had about the patients. They also collected the patients' postal codes and assigned a social deprivation score on the basis of the Jarman index. We then matched this anonymized material with the expenditure on each patient from the fund. This enabled us to see whether the practice could predict the kinds of patient that would be expensive and enabled us to see how far the DoH's formula would compensate the practice for the extra cost of predictably expensive patients.

## THE PRACTICES

We should like to give some flavour of our ten diverse practices but can only summarize a few characteristics and examples here.

There were three inner city practices in the sample – one in cramped premises in an affluent area with many young and transient patients; one, in a deprived area, had many orthodox Jews and an increasing number of refugees from Turkey, Kurdistan and Zaire – homeless or in hostels. The third, in an overcrowded health centre, had unusually elderly patients, but was developing a branch in a community centre on a new housing estate.

Both the two suburban and the five small town/semi-rural practices had more than one set of premises; sometimes three in different villages. Some were modern, some crowded, some spacious.

All the practices employed a wide range of staff. The smallest had three partners, most had between five and seven. A typical larger-practice staff included three nurses or nurse-practitioners, two medical secretaries, eight or more receptionists, a practice manager, one or more computer experts, two or three health visitors,

and maybe one or more part-time staff such as counsellors, physio-
therapists, a social worker, a dietician, a psychotherapist, an oph-
thalmologist, a rheumatologist – even a phlebotomist! District
nurses are often attached to the practices – and in some cases
dispensing plays an important role. Only one practice only had an
operating theatre – with four beds for local and general anaesthetic
surgery.

The second-wave practice was a small one in central London in an
area that was relatively affluent but was on the boundary of a much
poorer neighbourhood. It had a significant number of private
patients.

The third wave covered a much broader socio-economic and
geographical mix. We had a central London practice in a poor area,
one in an Outer London area with a mixed population, one on a
large outer London council housing estate, one in a New Town and
many in small towns with a full social mix. The better-off suburban
ring was less dominant than the first-wave group. Again there were
rural practices rather like some of those in our first wave. The
spread of fundholding was reflected in so far as we could match it in
our small sample.

# 4

# IMPLEMENTING THE SCHEME

## DRIVE FROM THE CENTRE

Until the Thatcher administration of the 1980s the British civil service's preferred style of implementation was to prepare a policy in as much detail as possible, thinking about all the possible pitfalls in advance, though not necessarily avoiding them. This minimized potential embarrassment for the minister and those charged with carrying out policy. But as we know from the experience of the Labour Government in the 1960s and 1970s, this could delay a piece of social legislation considerably.

Mrs Thatcher's style was different. Get the outline of a policy and force it through regardless, stop the civil service prevaricating and sort out the problems as you go along. The Poll Tax was the most obvious and disastrous example of this strategy. The NHS reforms of 1989–91 fit the same style.

The review of the National Health Service Mrs Thatcher had ordered was to report within 12 months. In the autumn of 1988 little hard progress had been made. Mrs Thatcher let it be known that she wanted a White Paper to be published at the end of that 12 months, come what may. This left little more than two months to settle the future of one of the largest and most popular social institutions in the country. As we have seen, the fundholding element was the least worked out. The White Paper contained only the very barest bones of the scheme. There was no clear definition of what procedures would be included or how the GPs' budgets would be set. Those charged with implementing the scheme would have to make up the rules of the game as they went along. Yet there had to be rules. This was not a case where front-line professionals could do things very differently in different parts of the country. Public money was being paid out in large amounts. Moreover, it was a highly visible policy. The Prime Minister was deeply involved. The Secretary of State himself was the particular champion of the whole idea. Civil servants could not afford it to fail. Nor, if they valued their future or their performance-related pay, could regional managers!

On the other hand, the NHS reforms were deeply unpopular. In 1990–2 it seemed as if they might lose the Government the looming election. GP fundholding turned out to be one of the most contentious elements in an unpopular package.

In these rather unusual circumstances, the civil servants most closely involved developed an innovative style of implementation that does not fit either the top-down blue print or the bottom-up local discretionary model discussed in Chapter 3.

Another analogy was to fit the events more closely. Charles Schultze (1968), of the Brookings Institution, once distinguished two kinds of planning: 'Cook's tour planning', where everyone knows exactly where they are going, and 'Lewis and Clark planning'. The American explorers, Lewis and Clark, were merely told to find a route to the Pacific. They did so by finding the watershed, following the rivers to the sea using their wits as they went.

The implementation of fundholding can be seen as a Lewis and Clark adventure – but in this instance there was telephonic contact between the field explorers and the equivalent of Washington and regular flights back to discuss progress with other explorers.

Each region had a GP fundholding development officer and contact person. These individuals kept in regular contact with the small team in the DoH charged with making fundholding work. At the outset there were just two people charged with getting the scheme going – a medical adviser who had been involved in the original idea in the mid-1980s and a young civil servant from outside the DoH who became an enthusiast. Both were looked on with some suspicion by traditionalist officials. They were in that rather remote part of the DoH that had dealt with the old Family Practitioner Committees. The newly-formed NHS Management Executive dealt directly with Regional Health Authorities and through them with District Health Authorities. It was primarily responsible for making district purchasing work. Fundholders were a distraction and a nuisance. What the two evangelists did have on their side, however, was ministerial, indeed Prime Ministerial, support. There are close parallels with an earlier very different reform – the creation of the Open University (Hall *et al.*, 1975). On that occasion, too, an unusual idea, treated with grave suspicion by the central department, was only carried through with Prime Ministerial support.

The civil servants began work in 1989, seeking to define much more closely what the boundaries of the scheme actually were. What surgical procedures would be in and what out? What would happen to patients referred for one treatment and then passed on by the consultant to another speciality? Who would pay? How exactly would the budgets be set? On what criteria should practices be chosen or rejected when they applied to join the scheme? How many practices did they want in the first wave?

One of the senior strategy groups in the DoH concerned with the NHS reforms worked on GP fundholding. Beneath that was the working group that met monthly, composed of all the regional fundholding officers and the DoH civil servants charged with implementation. This evolved into a two-way system of almost continuous interchange. The civil servants would tell the regional officers where they had got to in developing the detailed rules and hear the regional officers' reactions to their feasibility. Regional officers raised difficulties they were experiencing. These were often phoned in, in desperation, between meetings. The civil servants would come up with a rule and this would be faxed round the regional officers and discussed at the next monthly meeting. The civil servants also went to conferences of intending fundholders and made themselves very accessible. Thus, many of the keenest GPs would also be on the telephone to the DoH with their difficulties and angry reactions to delays or adjudications to which they objected. Some fundholding GPs had direct access to ministers.

All in all, this was a much more open and flexible way of implementing policy than any other the authors have observed. Yet policy made up 'on the hoof' is likely to leave untied ends and possible strategic problems patched but not solved. We shall return to that theme in later chapters. In what follows we describe a highly successful example of Lewis and Clark exploration. Sir John Simon (Lambert, 1963) would have been proud of his descendants!

The circumstances did not look propitious. The British Medical Association (BMA) had sworn its opposition. It pronounced the scheme doomed and wrote to all practices urging them not to participate (*The Times*, 1 June 1990). It predicted the development of a two-tier system and a split between GPs in and out of the system (*British Medical Journal*, April 1990). The Government's decision to enforce a 'contract' on GPs a year earlier had seriously soured the relationship between Government and family doctors. The DoH decided to communicate directly with GPs. Every GP was sent a simple, well-presented outline of the scheme, answering the kinds of immediate questions that a GP might have (*Funding General Practice: The Programme for the Introduction of General Practice Budgets*, January 1990). Almost universally the GPs we interviewed thought it was well done and informative.

At the back of the document was a list of the names and addresses and telephone numbers of one individual in each region who would be responsible for fundholding – the fundholding officer. This was a shrewd move. Regions were to be responsible for launching the scheme but GPs had never normally had any dealings with regions. The Family Practitioner Committees (FPCs), as they then were, were their only contact with NHS bureaucracy. These names gave a point of contact in a strange faceless organization.

Equally important there was a tear-off slip at the back of the document, which GPs could send in expressing a preliminary interest in joining the scheme 'without prejudice'. The regional officers would then be obliged to follow up all these expressions of intent.

The eligible list size was reduced from the originally announced 11,000 to 9000 because it was feared not enough practices would join.

There were also financial inducements. GPs joining the scheme would be given the costs of purchasing, leasing or upgrading a computer system needed to run the information side of fundholding. Moreover, in the preparatory year, an allowance would be paid to cover the extra administrative costs of preparing the practice for fundholding status. The precise arrangements followed a long dispute between GPs and the DoH. A management allowance would be paid to cover the costs of administering the fund when the practice joined the scheme and the full allowance would be paid from the first full year. All these were attempts to sell the idea to practices struggling to come to terms with the information demands of the new GP contract as well as this information-hungry scheme.

## REGIONS LAUNCH THE SCHEME

Because of the political importance of the scheme, Regional Health Authorities had to take the lead. The old Family Practitioner Committees were being transformed into Family Health Service Authorities (FHSAs), with new chief officers, and were deeply involved in administering the new contract with GPs. They were not yet in a position to take the lead. Moreover, as the fundholding GPs' budgets would be top sliced from the budgets the districts would get, regions had a strong interest in managing the pace of change and above all keeping a close eye on the size of those budgets. Just what the job would involve, however, no one knew.

The regional managers we spoke to in January 1990 really had no idea what to expect but they thought the response from GPs would be modest. 'Perhaps', one officer said, 'we might get as many as five or six practices applying.' Regions were in for a shock.

In one of our regions, Region B, 78 practices made initial enquiries, 58 of whom were eligible. In Region A, 58 did so, while in the third, where we had been told GPs were largely hostile to the scheme, 36 showed an interest. Some of these practices were under the 9000 limit but, even excluding these, considerable numbers remained eligible and interested. At least one regional officer thought many GPs had not fully considered the consequences and were opting into unknown territory with abandon.

Officers were worried. We certainly came across strong doubts about fundholding amongst managers within the service: it would upset the patient–doctor relationship, it was unrealistic for GPs to change their provider units, it was pointless complicating the funding arrangements in what was going to be a difficult year. GPs would have enough to do coping with the new contract and its organizational demands. A practice would have to be very well organized to take on both changes at the same time.

Managers at regional, district and FPC level, therefore, had good reason to be apprehensive of the large number of practices that had applied. Districts feared disruption to their budgets. On the other hand the DoH and ministers were making it clear that practices had a right to enter the scheme if they were fit to do so. If practices appealed over the heads of the region to the Secretary of State, he would probably uphold the GPs' right to join the scheme. The regions had a difficult course to steer in the preparatory year.

They did not want too many practices in the scheme, nor did they want to run foul of the DoH.

In England as a whole, 712 practices had applied by March 1990. The scheme would, at least, take off. Would it fly?

To initiate the changes outlined above, organizational changes were necessary at Regional Health Authority (RHA) level. Hitherto, general practice had had a marginal status in most RHAs. Even in the new situation GP fundholding was not high on their agenda. It was seen as a small part of a larger package of changes.

The regions in our study began with a single officer responsible for fundholding spending only part of his or her time on this initiative. In one case the individual was a GP acting as the Region's adviser on general practice matters. In Region B, with the highest number of interested practices – nearly 80 – more staff had to be assigned to the initiative. A second officer was appointed to act as the day-to-day link person, visiting the practices and explaining the scheme's detail – a facilitator. A full-time Family Practitioner Service Manager was appointed to take charge of what had become a large operation. In the region with the second largest expression of interest – Region A – the FPC Liaison Officer and Primary Care Development Officer found he was spending most of his time on GP fundholding. He was given an assistant to be the project manager for fundholding. In the third region, a full-time officer was appointed rather later and took over primary responsibility, leaving the GP adviser to revert to his original role as a professional adviser on general practice. Thus the regional input was larger than had been expected and varied depending on the scale of initial interest shown by practices. So, too, did the managerial style.

Region B adopted the most proactive role. It had a project team of officers including, in addition to the fundholding service manager and other senior managers, a finance officer, a medical officer and computing and statistical help. This group carried the process forward. The information required of the practices, the selection criteria, the budget-setting process, were all discussed by this group. It was felt that to include GPs or others in a representative capacity would involve a clash of interest.

Regional officers visited practices and drew up a profile of their strengths and limitations, drawing on FPC experience, before making an initial judgement. The selection was made relatively early compared to the other two regions. The information requested was detailed and defined quite quickly. Too quickly, officers agreed in retrospect.

The most common complaint from GPs was that the data collection needed to set the budgets had not been sufficiently discussed with GPs. One GP said, 'Expectations were far beyond what was needed. They used a sledgehammer to crack a nut. We sent in 1500 forms. They could have spent a week in the practice analysing our data at different times and reached the same conclusions.' Much of the information had to be extracted by hand. The problem for the Region was that practices' information systems were so diverse in kind and quality. They needed consistent returns to calculate the practices' budgets. The regional hospital activity information proved so unreliable it could not be used for setting budgets. More piloting and consultation with practices might have smoothed GPs' reactions but the time-scale was desperately short. As it was, regional officers felt that the data collected for budget setting had been inadequate.

Conferences and workshops were held for practices to inform them about fundholding. Budget presentations were made to each practice individually to explain how their budget had been calculated. The regional officer for fundholding and the regional financial officer for fundholding went through the budget line by line, answering questions and leaving the practices to respond. There then followed arguments with the practices about the data, the assumptions used and any unusual circumstances that might be affecting the practices' referrals in the period sampled. Nevertheless, the practices in this region seem to have understood the basis of the calculation rather well. They were fast learners in this school of accountancy.

As we shall see this proactive approach had both advantages and some initial problems. Given the high number of intending practices, an active response was needed, but the group of first-wave fundholders included a number of very articulate and independent practices who reacted badly to their first experience of regional involvement.

In Region A a consultative working group included the regional managers, FPC officers, a district general manager and some GPs. We were able to attend its meetings. A great deal of time was spent working out how to select which practices should be given fundholding status in the first year. The original intention was to use a

**Table 4.1**   Selection criteria for practices in Region A

---

*Reasons for considering fundholding*
The RHA and the FHSA would like to know why the practice considers
fundholding status would benefit the patients on the practice list. Practices may
identify several likely benefits to be derived from fundholding.

*Partnership commitment*
The RHA will need to be convinced that the practice has examined the workload
implications of fundholding; and the ways in which the responsibilities of operating
a fund will impinge on its work as clinicians. Whilst it is likely that not all partners
in a practice will be equally enthusiastic about the prospects of fundholding, the
RHA would need to be assured that there were no strong opponents; and that the
decision to prepare for fundholding would not prejudice the cohesion of the
partnership.

*Management arrangements*
In discussion with the partnership, the Region would like to identify how the
practice allocates administrative responsibilities at the moment; whether the
practice has a manager, and if so what is her/his remit; and the practice's view on
the enhancement it would need, in order to absorb the extra managerial workload.
The RHA will also be interested in the way a practice manages and controls
existing funds, and how the financial management is integrated with the rest of its
activities.

*Practice development plan*
The RHA group will be looking for evidence that a planning framework of some
sort, albeit perhaps less formally described, exists within the practice for looking at
future service developments. Evidence of taking forward new projects in the recent
past – becoming a training practice, for example; or a change in management
arrangement – may well be evidence of an ability for innovation in the future.

*Information and information technology*
The RHA will want to know whether the practice routinely collects information on
its referrals to hospital; whether the practice routinely monitors hospital waiting
time and waiting lists; and what information the practice routinely collects about
the population which it serves.

On computing, the Region will need any practice entering the scheme to be
adequately supported. At this stage, the RHA will wish to enquire whether the
practice has a full computer system now; how the system is integrated into the work
of the practice, and whether the system will require further enhancement for
fundholding. If the practice does not have an adequate system at the moment, the
RHA would need to be satisfied that the plans exist to acquire one and that the
space, staffing and (especially) the training implications are being examined.

*Support staff and premises*
Practices aiming for fundholding should be aware of any support staff requirement,
particularly for budget management and computer support, and have given some
thought as to how these might be met. The RHA will pay heed to the standards of
the current building, space within them to expand clinical and management
activities, and whether any major moves or building works are planned – and how
these might affect preparatory work on fundholding.

---

quantitative measure of practice characteristics, at least to show that the decisions had not been purely judgemental. In the end this proved not to be feasible. The criteria that were adopted are set out in Table 4.1. They were not that different from those used in other regions. A lot of time was taken in an attempt to be objective. Many practices dropped out in that time, leaving a modest number entering the scheme in the first year – a result with which the regional officers were not unhappy!

Region C took the view from the outset that, as far as possible, the administration of the scheme should be left to the FHSAs. The practices in the scheme were largely concentrated in one FHSA. It handled most of the practical issues except budget setting. The GPs seemed barely aware of Region's role, except to fix the budget, which had been done in a fairly relaxed way.

In every case the regions had to move fundholding up their agenda. In one case this was made more necessary by the results of a management game that were widely reported in the national press. This was a three-day simulation game of the possible outcome of an internal market. Players were assigned roles as purchasers and providers. While relative calm prevailed in year one, after this wide variations, and indeed possible financial collapse, ensued as the players became more aggressive in their competitive strategies. So much was reported. It was less widely appreciated that it was the fundholding practices that caused the biggest potential changes. After this, fundholding came to have a higher profile with senior regional management.

Thus, regions had begun by seeing fundholding as a rather small element in the whole reform package. They soon recognized that a significant regional input was required. In areas where a large number of practices participated the new FHSAs came to provide a supportive role (see below). However, the capacity and interest in fundholding exhibited by FHSAs at this point varied widely. Some were outright opponents of the whole idea, often reflecting local GP opinion.

### The practices flex their collective muscle

In June 1990 the practices in two counties met together and discussed their mutual problems. A letter was written to the Chairman of the RHA objecting to the way the scheme was being implemented by regional officers. The GPs concerned were worried by the quantity of information that was being demanded by the Region about their practices. Some information, it was thought, transgressed the confidential nature of the patient–doctor relationship, such as the number of private patients; other information on referrals should be obtained from provider units, they argued.

They claimed they were among the most successful, businesslike and efficient practices in the country. They objected to being asked to provide business plans, and the heavy demands for information, many thought to be unnecessary, placed extra burdens on already 'hard-pressed' doctors. The request by Region to put the bulk of that information on a paper-based system of returns was unacceptable, particularly in view of the high standards of computer efficiency required by the Region before participation was agreed. Criticisms were also made of the design of that system and the period for sampling referral data. The hundreds of hours spent by GPs on the fundholding initiative were not being reimbursed under the management allowance, they claimed. The letter ended with a request that these matters should receive urgent attention, or the GPs concerned would have to reconsider their positions as potential fundholders.

The Regional Chairman replied two weeks later, beginning with praise for the quality of general practice in the Region. He thought that the presumed distrust and confrontation with regional officers referred to was a misunderstanding of the spirit of hard work that had gone into setting up the initiative.

It was agreed that there should be a review of the minimum data set. He assured GPs that there was no wish to add to the workload, and managers would be very willing to discuss business plans and work programmes with individual practices.

It was reaffirmed that GPs could not be reimbursed for additional work. Certain tasks had to remain the responsibility of the RHAs, most importantly the policy development, but the management process would increasingly be left to the FPCs. It was agreed that fundholding meetings could be recognized for expenses.

These protests became public, and featured in the medical press. The Government and the Region gave some ground, for example, on the range of information requested from practices.

This series of exchanges illustrated how GPs could rapidly find a collective voice to articulate their interests. There was some discussion of forming a breakaway fundholders' union, breaking away from the BMA, which was still hostile to fundholding. In the end the prime movers in this episode set up a national association of fundholders that acted as a pressure group and information exchange, not a rival to the BMA. The large number of GPs in these two FPCs gave them substantial political muscle, which they were prepared to use to effect change. This collective response resulted in a loose but more long-term local group forming. GPs for the first time, as fundholders, found they had a unified voice, which, once raised, could influence policy.

Groups emerged in other areas where there were several practices. They met regularly to discuss common issues, to compare notes on prices and contracts that providers were offering and on what the Region was doing. They later offered support to the second- and third-wavers who joined the scheme. In one rural area the fundholders met to give each other mutual support in the first instance. There was a lot of hostility from other GPs and sharing problems with sympathetic GPs was a help. After this initial period the meetings were used to discuss a common approach to contracting. They also provided a forum for meeting the providers and consultants. Details were left to networking. 'All the practice managers are always on the phone to one another. If anything new comes up faxes flash between them', as one partner put it.

As Weiner and Ferriss (1990) predicted from American experience, networks emerged to strengthen the practices' political and purchasing power.

### The geographical spread

A combination of factors affected who applied to enter the scheme in the first wave: the practices had to be well managed, to have an established, computerized patient database, the partners had to have spare time and energy, there had to be space to house the extra staff needed. This restricted the type of practice that could apply. The fairly demanding selection procedure also meant that there was an uneven spread of practices entering fundholding in the first year. The highest concentration lay in suburban areas.

## REGIONS DEVOLVE DAY-TO-DAY ADMINISTRATION

It was clear that the regions' role as midwife would have to change as the number of practices joining the scheme grew. It would be impractical for regional officers to visit each intending practice, nurse them through the early stages and negotiate each budget individually. FHSAs were the front line agencies responsible for relations with GPs and they should add this function to their list of responsibilities. Yet regions also felt they could not let go of certain key aspects of the scheme.

First and foremost was the question of the budget. There had been a lot of criticism from district health authority managers and chief officers of the way the regions had set the first-wave practices' budgets. It was felt they had been too generous and that districts had had too much sliced from their budgets. Each of the regions wanted to keep a tight hold on the methodology used to set practices' target allocations and to monitor the outcomes closely. On the other hand, the DoH showed some displeasure at the slow progress of fundholding in two of the regions, and officers felt the need to encourage some FHSAs to be more active in recruiting practices.

In year two of the scheme the two regions with a large role in phase one devolved the task of direct contact with practices almost entirely to FHSAs. The region with most fundholders reduced from two to one the number of staff responsible for the scheme plus specialist support. Negotiation with intending practices was left to the FHSAs working within the guidelines agreed. Support and advice to individual practices was the FHSA's responsibility. So, too, was the monitoring of the budget spend, with the region to be alerted if any practice was straying significantly into surplus or deficit. Regions did, however, tighten the budget-setting rules. One region took a very active role in reviewing past budgets and working towards formula funding. We discuss this in Chapter 9.

The administration of the second-wave entry went far more smoothly than the first wave. The practices got on with filling in the data sheets that told the FHSAs where they had referred patients, with little complaint. With some exceptions the budgets were set with little acrimony.

The third-wave practices were much more relaxed about the whole procedure. Some said they did not get much help from their FHSA officers, who often knew little about fundholding, but they did get help from practice managers from the first-wave group who had been through it all before.

In two of our regions the third wave, although much larger than the previous waves, went through relatively smoothly in the de-centralized way begun the previous year.

The third of our regions faced a more difficult time. It already had one of the largest proportions of the population under fundholders' care of any region. The third wave was large. Moreover, in one particular county nearly two-thirds of the population were in fund-holding practices. As in another region in similar circumstances, the districts were concerned. They felt they were losing control of the services covered by fundholding. They argued that they could not afford to do elective surgery any more. The demands of emergency work meant that they had to keep reducing the share of their budget they could allocate to non-emergency care. Fundholders, whose budgets were fixed on the basis of historic levels of elective surgery, were exempt from this squeeze. Their budgets were sliced from the district budget leaving districts even less to give their hospitals to cover the costs of elective surgery for non-fundholding patients. The districts complained bitterly that they and non-fundholding patients were being discriminated against and that the system of financing fundholders was grossly unfair.

Region decided to embark on a major review of the impact of fundholding and to ask for outside help in designing a basis of formula funding that would test whether fundholders were out of line and set budgets that put them on an equivalent basis. We discuss this in Chapter 9. It once more put the Region on a confrontational course with practices. A more gradual move to the Region's new targets was finally accepted. The whole episode illustrated the key importance of the budget-setting process and how difficult it will be for regions to keep out of it, at least before some automatic formula can be worked out.

## THE ROLE OF FHSAs

In 1990 when we first visited the FHSAs in our regions they were still coming to terms with their change from being FPCs. We looked at four in particular. Three had reappointed the old FPC managers to be chief executives; one had introduced an outsider. Each set up a small team of officers to oversee the fundholding project. Most managers thought that few practices would be in a position to cope with a budget of the size contemplated and would not have the time or energy to do so given the complaints there had been about the work involved in the new contract. They thought they would have to keep a careful watch on the practices' financial capacity. They had little or no idea what role FHSAs would be called on to play. In one area 60 per cent of the practices had more than the minimum 9000 patients. Fifty-four practices qualified and 13 joined in the first round. The FHSA decided to go with the flow. The practices formed themselves into a loose consortium and one of the managers in the FHSA took on the responsibility of contracting with hospitals on behalf of ten of these 13. This gave him very considerable leverage. He was able to offer considerable custom to hospitals who wanted to make special deals on costly items. He advocated the use of cost and volume contracts with the main local hospitals from the outset, holding back from contracting the whole budget to give practices some leverage over providers. He had the time to monitor contracts regularly. He could negotiate cost per case treatments with specialist hospitals. The practices welcomed his expertise as well as the greater bargaining power he gave them. Here was an FHSA manager strengthening the hand of GPs. Moreover, he was able to cross district boundaries, organizing as he did, GPs from three districts. The GPs decided which hospitals they wanted to use and the FHSA facilitator and contract manager tried to obtain the best deal for that practice. The FHSA suggested going even further and acting as a combined budget-holder for all the GPs. This was rejected by the GPs. Later this individual was to become a private consultant to fundholders. This proactive stance by the FHSA helped sustain the fundholders and pushed the whole process forward.

The FHSA thought the districts had misjudged fundholding initially, presuming that it would simply go away.

Another of the FHSAs we looked at had also taken a very supportive and interventionist role but was rebuffed to some extent by the first-wave fundholders, who preferred to keep their independence and run their own fundholding group, setting their own contracts and working closely together. At the other extreme some FHSAs were deeply suspicious of fundholding and essentially against it in principle for the divisive effects they thought it would have.

Like it or not, in year two, and even more in year three, FHSAs became front-line administrators of the scheme. Again their attitudes varied. Some put fairly junior people in post as fundholding liaison officers. The GPs soon realized they would do far better to seek advice from first-wavers or the local group. In other areas fundholding became the major preoccupation of the FHSA, who set up good databases and close monitoring of budgets. The FHSA became the defender of fundholders when they came under attack, moderating the regions' demands for immediate major cuts in fundholders' budgets. They sought to build better understanding between the district health authorities and fundholders.

In 1993 the Audit Commission reviewed the work of FHSAs nationally and its report, *Practices Make Perfect*, describes the whole range of monitoring and accountability tasks they have to perform far beyond looking after fundholders (Audit Commission, 1993a). Only about one page of the report covers their fundholding responsibilities. The report comments on the wide variations in budgets between practices and on cases of 'unrealistic budget setting and/or changes in referral patterns that had produced surpluses in excess of £100,000 in 40 cases'. As we have seen, these had more to do with regions' difficulties in budget setting than with FHSAs.

## OVERVIEW

We began by characterizing the implementation of GP fundholding as a Lewis and Clark mission of exploration. Did the explorers find the Pacific? The answer is that they did but they have not yet secured the territory.

In terms of sheer improvisation and speed those responsible must be given very nearly full marks. The trail they blazed with the first-wave fundholders has been followed by more practices than ever seemed possible when we began interviewing in January 1990. The scheme began with the outright opposition of the BMA. By the end of the project, in the summer of 1993, the BMA had withdrawn its in-principle opposition. Most eligible practices were now either in the scheme or signing up to join later waves.

Considering how limited the original ground plan was the practical detail put in place in the three years has also been impressive, especially since the scope of the scheme was extended significantly in 1992, just before the general election, to include community health services in the budget.

However, the exploratory nature of the quest and the improvisations have also left their legacy. If, as some argued at the outset, the scheme had been confined to a small group of innovative practices acting as efficiency advocates and irritant pioneers, the districts might have accepted them as part useful, part irrelevant, actors. They would not have been threats to the very existence of districts. Yet the very success of fundholding began to call the future of districts into question. In the county with the largest number of fundholders, the three districts and the FHSA joined to form a single purchasing agency – a direct response to the scale of the fundholders' purchasing capacity and influence. The incremental growth of fundholding required a reassessment of existing authorities' boundaries and functions of both districts and FHSAs. In early 1993 the Secretary of State for Health announced the appointment of a review group to consider yet again the structure and responsibilities of regions, districts and FHSAs (Ham, 1993b; Higgins, 1993). Late in 1993 the Secretary of State proposed to amalgamate regions and move towards abolishing them as a separate tier of authority. Just who would administer the GP fundholders was less than clear.

The second main piece of unfinished business concerned the setting of budgets. Fixing budgets on the basis of past referral patterns had been a temporary expedient. It was proving difficult to move on to a formula that would be fair to fundholders and non-fundholders alike. We discuss the issues in detail in Chapter 9.

Some regions were experimenting with extending the scope of the fundholders' budgets. The Labour Party was still advocating the end of the scheme. The reforms seemed to be the beginning of more change, not the prelude to stability.

# 5

# WHAT DID THE PRACTICES HOPE TO ACHIEVE?

From a popular television series (*Peak Practice*) and much press comment, one might deduce that GPs wish to become fundholders for a mixture of two motives – to make money and to get better services for their patients at the expense of others.

We spent many of our earliest interviews with practices discussing why they had chosen to become fundholders; we asked the third-wavers the same thing. We asked the first-wave practices three and a half years after we first saw them what they thought they had achieved.

Over the period of the research good relations were established, in which discussions became very frank about the GPs' motives and tactics, financial and professional. Wherever possible we took note of others' perceptions of what was going on, such as NHS managers who knew the practices well, and we checked the plausibility of the accounts against the actions of the practices, matching stated intentions against what actually happened. Our sample was not likely to include those with the most to hide, but our regional officers all said that the practices we had chosen were, in their view, a fair cross-section of the scheme at both stages. We cannot do more than claim that the account that follows is as fair as we can make it in those circumstances.

## FIRST-WAVERS' INTENTIONS

### Improving quality of service

In all the nearly four years of interviewing we have done it is impossible not to conclude that improving the quality of the service practices could give was the GPs' primary objective. All the first-wave practices used this phrase, or something like it, to describe their motivation. When pressed, most described some aspect of their local hospital service with which they were unhappy, frequently waiting times or a poor speciality with a particularly unhelpful consultant. None wanted to move all their patients but most had at least one or two specialities they wished to change or threaten in order to improve matters. Some of the most passionate advocates of the new scheme were also passionately pro-NHS. They saw the scheme as a way of shaking up a highly ineffective hospital system. As one put it, 'This is the NHS's last chance for me. If it does not come off I shall leave the profession.' This young GP threw himself into the scheme and was a source of continual, if sometimes resented, pressure on local providers. Other practices had been in a less advantageous market position and expressed some disappointment, after three years, at what they had managed to achieve, but their own assessments of the scheme still reflected this initial concern to improve hospital service quality. Most put 'changed attitudes by the hospital' or some similar phrase at the top of their list of achievements.

### Referral freedom

About three-quarters of the practices in 1990 had been very concerned that, under the new district purchasing arrangements, their district would not permit them to send patients to hospitals of their choice outside the district. They believed districts would make contracts with only one or two providers and severely restrict their freedom to refer. For them it was the prime motive for joining the scheme. They wanted to retain the freedom they had always had to refer where they wished. The capacity to pay the receiving hospital cash for their patients would ensure this freedom, they felt.

### Service developments in the practice

Slightly fewer, but still a majority, were keen to provide more on-site services, mostly counselling and physiotherapy, for example, but only three of the ten at this early stage had the idea that consultants might come and do outpatient clinics, and two wanted to do minor operations. Their ambitions were modest at this point. As we shall see, this aspect of the scheme developed in years one and two of the scheme, as ideas travelled fast in the fundholding network.

## Budgetary freedom

All looked forward to having a staff budget they could spend as they wished without having to ask the FHSA's permission to employ staff. One practice later said that if nothing else had been achieved this had made the scheme worth while. Several said in our last interviews that 'being in control' had been a very important gain and a large part of that was having budgetary freedom over staff and the capacity to switch budgets between headings.

## Money and computing

Some of the practices were attracted by the idea that there might be some financial inducements, at least for the early waves, in joining the scheme. The opportunity the scheme might offer to get additional computing facilities was mentioned by half the original group. There were some cynics. One of the original sample of 15 who then dropped out said, 'The scheme has got to work. So the Government will bribe people in. We might as well pick up what is going.'

Some remarks were made about 'the small minority of greedy sharks who are giving fundholding a bad name'. Yet it soon became clear that there was not going to be much financial gain. The management allowance did enable practices to employ a manager and that benefited the whole practice. On the other hand, at least one partner had to spend a lot of time getting the scheme off the ground, learning about the details, considering if not doing the contracting, attending conferences. Other partners had to take on more patients. There was plenty of private work or extra clinics, paid for under the new contract, that the practices might have been doing and which would have paid much better. Fundholding could be a distraction from things that would have increased partners' own income. In these early stages the idea of GPs forming themselves into private companies to purchase from themselves (see Chapter 2) had not been invented and none of our practices felt they would be able to make large savings on their budgets. The fear was the reverse. The main financial worry was that they would run out of budget early in the year and not be able to get their patients treated.

It soon became obvious to all in our sample who remained in the scheme that they had better do so for non-financial reasons. As one partner put it to us, 'Anyone who thinks they are going to make money out of this needs their head examining.'

## The next mountain

For most in the first wave the scheme was seen as the thing any leading practice in an area should seek to do. It was 'the wave of the future'. Many were teaching practices, they had made all the improvements in the practice organization they could. Ordinary general practice had become something of a routine. The interest and excitement came from doing new things, expanding and improving the practice premises, helping educate student doctors, installing a new computerized patient record system, running specialist clinics. All our sample had been innovators in one or all of these ways. They were not, mostly, borne down with coping with an inner-city practice, though some had deprived populations. They had the 'entrepreneurial space' to experiment. All were well run and were eager to do new things for their patient populations. This scheme seemed to offer the freedom and incentives to do that. This was the next mountain to climb.

While main-line NHS managers were not enthusiastic about competition and market reforms, these GPs were more at home with the notion. 'We are already running a business', one said, 'which is more than these regional officers have ever done.' 'We are already in the market place,' said one practice manager, with several competing practices on the door step, 'we attract patients or go out of business.'

GP partnerships are a joint business enterprise and the financial health of the practice has always been a significant part of GPs' concerns. This may explain why some GPs took to the idea of a competitive market more easily than NHS managers did. They adapted to notions of purchasing and contracting more quickly than the hospitals with whom they were seeking to do business.

## WORRIES

Balancing these hopes were a set of very worrisome concerns. The major ones expressed in these early interviews were, the administrative load the scheme would bring the practice, the capacity of the computer system to cope (indeed whether one would exist at all) and the uncertainties about being able to handle the budget and keep within it.

Those who expressed interest and did *not* join, and those we interviewed who opposed the whole idea, had other worries. One fear expressed by most of the opponents was that the scheme would introduce a financial element into their relations with their patients. They would have to take account of the possible cost of their recommended referral or drug prescription. They might be tempted to delay treatment. Even though they might not give way to such considerations they were afraid their patients would *think* they were being affected by such factors.

One of the most interesting contrasts to emerge in this first round of interviews with joiners and non-joiners was the different attitude to rationing. Two thoughtful opponents of the scheme said they recognized that the NHS had to ration services, it was an inevitable consequence of being in a tax-financed system. Someone had to say 'no' or 'join the queue' but they would much rather the hospital consultant did that. They did not want to be a party to making such decisions, telling one patient they had a lower priority than another patient. It would break the patient's trust and was not part of a GP's job.

The fundholders tended to take a very different professional view. It was well expressed by one fundholder, who also agreed that rationing was necessary, but said:

> I am the best judge of my patients' need. Let's face it, who gets seen first in a hospital is pretty arbitrary. It often amounts to what the consultant's secretary picks off the pile first. I know my patients well. I know if this one does not get his operation soon he will never work again and he has a family to keep, or her marriage will break up. There is no way a consultant can know that sort of thing. If I have to take those decisions they will be better just because I know more about the individual cases.

By the time we conducted our later interviews in June 1991 this view had gained ground amongst those who had opted into the scheme. Districts were taking relatively little notice of GP priorities in their contracting, at least as the GPs saw it, and this reinforced the view that they would like to have a direct say in the rationing criteria that would affect their own patients.

We asked how far practices had involved patients in the decision to become fundholders.

None of the practices had consulted their patients when they decided to apply to enter the scheme. GPs looked on this stage as if it were an examination of the practice or a job application. It was a very hot issue politically. A mixture of reasons were given for not consulting. When fundholding status had been agreed the practices did tell their patients in a number of different ways. Most simply left leaflets about in the waiting room or put a notice up and answered questions if patients raised them. Very few did ask, we were told.

Some practices went to greater lengths. One called a village meeting, described the scheme, answered questions and a lively discussion followed. Another sent an invitation to a one in three sample of the practice population and asked them to come to meetings in the practice. After a general talk the partners split the audience into groups and discussed the issues more informally, one GP per group.

Some public anger was generated in one area that fundholding status had not been discussed with patients.

## INTENTIONS AND OUTCOMES

In the months leading up to April 1991 a number of practices lost heart and nearly gave up. The hostility of local colleagues, 'more bitter than I have experienced on any other professional issue', was part of it. Most difficult was the refusal of the providers to have anything to do with them and the uncertainty and lateness of the contracting process. Uncertainty about the rules of the game, computing and budget setting added to the frustration. There have been subsequent periods of pessimism, for example, when one region tried to cut their budgets substantially in the third year. The scheme has taken more time and energy than they expected for longer.

Yet, in mid-1993, morale was high. When we asked our sample about the balance sheet all thought the scheme had been a success. Most thought it was *the* model for the future of the NHS. All thought it had made the hospitals more responsive to general practice. Many thought the budget should be extended to the whole of hospital care and a few argued that social service provisions for community care should be included. The complaints were of restrictions to the scheme and what they saw as attempts by regions and the DoH to claw back the freedoms the scheme had given them. The refusal of the DoH to relax the controls on community service contracts in 1993–4 was particularly irksome.

One of the unexpected side-effects mentioned by several practices was that it had brought the practice into the main stream of the health service for the first time. Contacts with managers of the local hospital had never happened on a serious level before. Serious discussions about local service issues with other GPs had begun with fundholding. 'We're part of the service now, we never were before.' This was a particularly interesting comment because it flies in the face of the common perception, and indeed our own initial predictions, but it was a general view.

In the autumn of 1992, and on to July 1993, we interviewed 16 third-wave practices on the same basis as the first-wavers and covered the same range of topics, at least initially. We also asked why the practices in our third-wave sample had not joined the first wave.

## Eligibility

About one-third of the practices had not been eligible before the size limit had been dropped. A few had been keen to join in the first place and jumped at the chance when the size limit was dropped. For most of the others there had been reservations two years earlier.

## Uncertainty

Many had felt the scheme had had an uncertain political future and were not sure how it would work. As one said, 'We wanted to see how it shook down before we committed ourselves.'

## Peer support

Some had been put off by the hostility of other GPs in the area. The emergence of local groups of fundholders, encouragement and advice from first-wavers and the existence of a national association of fundholders had tipped the balance with several practices.

### Ethical and political concerns

About one-quarter of the sample had had major ideological doubts about fundholding, or several members of the practice had. They felt it would produce a two-tier service and supporting it would be ethically unsound. As we had found two years earlier, there had been the fear that it would threaten the relationship with patients.

### No problems with providers

Another group had simply had no great motivation, feeling satisfied with their local providers.

### The costs of change

The fear of more organizational change had put off most of the other practices. In particular, many felt their computer systems were not up to the change. The fundholding option had come just about the time they were getting used to the new contract and they had felt that was quite enough change for the time being. Others had been going through a difficult patch in their practice, with new partners, and did not want to add to the strains.

For most it was a mixture of these reasons that had put them off the scheme in 1990 and 1991.

### Why did they join?

The problems had gradually come to seem less important. Local fundholders seemed to be coping without any great difficulty. The positive reasons had grown in weight and were drawn from watching the experience of the first two waves. Whatever the general objections to a two-tier service, they could not keep their patients from the benefits nor let the practice become less attractive. One of our practices described in some detail how it had made its decision. They thought of themselves as one of the most innovative health centres in the area and were strongly pro-NHS. They had decided when the reforms were announced that they wanted to have nothing to do with fundholding. They had never rethought that position or questioned it. Early in 1992 they went away for their annual retreat to think about the future of the practice. Fundholding was not on the agenda. They discussed the way they thought primary health care should go and what developments they would like to see happen: closer links with community services, doing more things on site, having a bigger say in certain specialities, especially the way the local psychiatric service was run. Having done this they realized that these were all things they could achieve, or were more likely to be achieved, in fundholding than outside. 'We decided, there and then to join the scheme.'

To a substantial extent the reasons given by the 16 third-wavers for joining the scheme mirrored those given by the first-wavers, but there was a different emphasis and the reasoning was based on watching the impact of the scheme locally rather than hope or theory.

**Service improvements**

Third-wavers all said they had seen how the first-wavers had made the local hospitals respond and take notice. First-wavers were perceived to be getting a more responsive service. Most felt this and thought their patients would be disadvantaged in the long run if they did not join. 'It was amazing', one said. 'Once the local providers heard we were going for fundholding they were on the phone. Never taken a blind bit of notice before.' One doctor said that rather than being a 'personal advocate' on behalf of some of his patients, especially the more articulate, he would rather be 'a purchasing advocate' for all his patients.

About one-quarter of our sample had been purchasing advisers to their district health authority. They felt frustrated that the GP's voice was not adequately heard. The process was slow and there was little feedback. The DHA was too heavily influenced by the providers to have a truly independent purchasing strategy. Fundholding would give them the chance to define their own requirements. As was evident from the interviews, there was considerable variety in what the practices wanted. They sought to 'fine tune' the district's contracts to their own practices' needs. What was different about the third wave was that they had had a chance to compare the first-wavers' contracts with the district's. They thought they could do better than the district too.

Many had also seen the extent to which first- and second-wavers were using their budgetary freedom to develop the range of services provided on their own premises. This was attractive and again they were anxious not to be left behind.

### Referral freedom

This featured less in the third-wave interviews, but half of those interviewed felt strongly that their district had limited the scope of the hospitals they could use. Many wanted to use their freedom to shop around and find shorter waiting times. One had been outraged by the fact that the district had run out of extra-contractual funds half-way through the year. He had always referred a few special cases to the regional teaching hospital and a letter telling him he could not do so for the next six months had so infuriated him, he persuaded his colleagues to apply.

### Consultants' private interests

One rather disturbing issue came up directly in several discussions and had never been aired as openly in the first-wave interviews. This was frustration with consultants who had private clinics and long waiting lists. In the GPs' view they were not trying as hard as they might to reduce waiting lists because long waits only encouraged patients to opt for private care.

### Future of general practice

Most felt that fundholding was now the future for primary health care, extending its scope. They had come to believe fundholding was here to stay. It was important for them to be in the forefront of general practice, especially if they were teaching trainee GPs.

### Optimum time to apply

Most thought that this was the best time to join the scheme. They would not have to face the problems the first-wave pioneers had faced. Fundholding was still relatively new, however, and there would still be financial inducements like computing.

### Budgetary freedom

Several practices said that being free of petty staffing controls and simply having a cash-limited budget was worth joining for on its own. Several were in areas where the local hospital had run out of cash for elective surgery cases three months before the end of the year; they had seen their waiting lists increase. They knew their fundholding colleagues had managed things better. They also wanted to be able to transfer money to develop services like counselling or community nursing, and felt that money was being wasted on hospital services.

## The next mountain

The number of sheer mountain climbers was less than in the first wave. There were fewer idealists, more hard-headed pragmatists learning from the gains and problems of the first- and second-wavers. There was little evidence of a general decline in the competence of the practices in managerial terms, indeed most were *better* prepared than the first-wavers at the same stage. There was a small tail, however, who needed a lot more support. Regional and FHSA officers claimed that this was even more true of the fourth-wavers.

## Calculating the balance sheet

For most practices the decision to enter fundholding had been more difficult than for the first-wave enthusiasts. Practices knew it would be time-consuming. They went to great lengths to weigh up the advantages and disadvantages. What else could they be doing with their time? One was still undecided when the deadline for joining was reached but decided that as the practice had invested so much effort already they would go ahead. On the other hand, many of the practices commented on the unexpected spin-offs from the process, even before they were operational. They had upgraded their patient computer software, they had had to make a detailed study of their referrals, which they had never done before, assuming they knew. They felt this had been worth while in itself. They now knew more about what was happening to their patients and what was happening in the practice. Partners had to share more information and concerns. They now knew more about how the community services worked. For the first time they knew which patients were receiving these services. There was much more they needed to find out but it had begun to make them think seriously about these services and what they wanted from them. Some thought it had brought the practice together instead of each GP working almost independently with their separate list of patients. Others argued that GPs had, since the NHS began, become deskilled, merely referral agencies. Now there would be opportunity to do more themselves, to run more services from the practice, to get consultants to visit the practice for outpatient clinics. Consultants were keen to both 'treat and teach' in the practice and this opened up the possibility of keeping abreast of new research and treatments. Many were keen to do more day surgery and to do the follow-up work themselves.

**Pressure from a new generation**

As one of the senior partners in one practice explained, the younger generation of GPs who were driving the reform on in his practice had joined general practice at a time when it was the first choice amongst a majority of the top medical students. They were very able. Some had opted out of the hospital when they had reached registrar status. They both knew their medicine and were critical of hospitals and especially of the follow-up care they knew their patients were getting. They wanted to change general practice and make it more interesting.

**Patient consultation**

The third-wave practices were more aware of the need to handle patient opinion carefully. Most external comment had been unfavourable to fundholding, they felt. Patients might feel they would not be treated if they cost too much and be affected by political attacks. So patients were informed the practice was to become fundholding through a newsletter. Practice staff were briefed to answer questions and allay fears. One practice received a long letter from a prominent member of the community complaining about going fundholding. They sent a long reasoned reply and the individual wrote back thanking them for explaining and accepting their reasons. There were instances of patients saying they would go elsewhere if the practice did not go fundholding. But all in all the practices had faced very little comment or interest.

One practice had set up a patient-participation group, selecting patients from each of the partners' lists. The purpose of the group was to help the practice with issues that fundholding might raise about purchasing or what developments were needed. It was hoped to develop its activities in the future.

## FIRST- AND THIRD-WAVERS COMPARED

Perhaps the most striking thing about the interviews with the third-wavers was their confidence and the extent to which the process had become routine. Many of the teething problems of the first wave had been sorted out. There were fewer complaints about the information demands or the rules of the game.

There was little comment about the Regional Health Authority's role. Since the first wave, regional officers had withdrawn, leaving day-to-day relations with the new practices in the scheme to FHSAs.

Many of the practices felt that the FHSAs lacked experience and often knew less than they did, given the help they had received from the first-wave practice managers in the area and from fundholders' meetings. However, most had good existing links with the senior FHSA managers and valued this.

The greatest help for the practice managers was derived from personal links with their first-wave counterparts, who often had let them spend days observing and learning the detailed nuts and bolts of the scheme. This was most true in the county areas outside London. There was much more confidence about contracting, a major worry to first-wavers. It had been done before, there were plenty of examples to use. The practices, in short, were relaxed about the practicalities and confident in their capacity to cope.

The second general characteristic that struck us was the more ambitious goals that had developed for the system in the two-year period. We have noted already the more extensive range of in-house services and consultants working from the practices. There were other examples. One group formed an alliance with most other GPs in the area and all were entering fundholding with the intention of seeking to preserve services in the local hospital, which the District wanted to close. Their plan was to contract with the hospital and essentially supply the funds needed to provide day surgery and other facilities they felt it important to keep as local as possible. Their patients were most unhappy at the prospect of having to travel for everything. They had won a lot of local support.

The enlarged fundholding groups were identifying commonly felt deficiencies in local provider services and were drawing up local agendas for action. Joint negotiations were envisaged for some services. One practice was negotiating with three others to open the local hospital operating theatre on a Saturday morning. Others were joining forces to create enough outpatient demand to justify a consultant coming to give sessions for three surgeries. All of this was more ambitious and more co-operative in tone than we had heard in the first round of interviews three and a half years earlier.

Just how far they and the first-wavers managed to fulfil these objectives we discuss in the following chapters.

# 6

# CONTRACTING: GPs OR DISTRICTS?

## THE THEORY OF CONTRACTING

At the heart of the NHS reforms was the belief that it would be beneficial to separate the functions of purchasing and providing and for purchasers to make contracts with competing providers.

### Supply-side inefficiency

The above belief derived in its turn from the economist's view that monopolistic providers, in any market, will tend to reap super-normal profits, exploiting consumers who have no power of exit (Hirschman, 1970). Producer domination in bureaucratic, non-profit organizations manifests itself not as monetary gain but in the form of '$X$-inefficiencies'. An example might be a consultant being consistently late, rarely turning up, leaving the job to juniors, not reducing a long waiting list. Equally, the hospital as a whole could be lax, with poor record-keeping, slow replies to letters and rude-ness and sloth by clerical staff.

Our interviews over the three years have convinced us that, though not universal, such lapses were all too common. This was not a strictly scientific conclusion, but the strength of feeling, the detailed examples given and the fact that they were often corroborated in independent interviews, reinforced this view. However, it would be wrong to suggest that such inefficiency was universal. Why not if monopoly was? The explanation probably lies in the crudity of the original theoretical model. First, professional staff are not only motivated by crude and short-term self-interest (Dunleavy, 1991). Saving lives, and improving patients' lot and comfort, bring their own reward. Second, professional staff move in a separate competitive market place. They are seeking jobs in other hospitals and, in their youth, at least, are anxious to be seen to be performing well. Third, the direct possibility of translating inefficiency into financial gain, by encouraging patients to go private, only occurs in some neighbourhoods and in some specialities. Thus, at one end of the spectrum we have young doctors with reputations to make or consolidate, working in situations that bring considerable professional satisfaction and with little opportunity to run a private clinic. At the other, we have older consultants stuck in a rather repetitive job, with a private clinic in a rich area. It is here that the worst abuses will occur, our modified theory predicts. Evidence from our interviews certainly fitted this hypothesis.

Nevertheless, competition will only produce efficiency gains when certain fairly tough conditions are met (Culyer and Posnett, 1990). There must be real competition between suppliers, the capacity for purchasers to opt for an alternative. There must be good information about quality and outcomes. Yet, as we argued in Chapter 1, purchasers of health care are in a relatively weak position to know about the productive efficiency of the hospitals they are purchasing from. Purchasers also need incentives to use what information they have and to contract in the best interests of their populations or members. If they are in a monopsonist situation and their 'customers' have no choice of purchaser, what incentive do these purchasers have to take their populations' interests into account?

**Demand-side diversity**

Monopoly purchasers have an interest in keeping the trouble of contracting to a minimum, not changing providers, establishing personal and friendly working relations with providers and making 'sweetheart contracts'. Districts are monopolist purchasers by definition, while GPs, in theory, are in competition for patients. This certainly varies geographically and is limited by the sheer inertia of patients. Yet there is, undoubtedly, contestability in the market for patients. This is supported by the evidence of our third-wave interviews where 'keeping ahead of the game' was a major motive for new joiners. Some Swedish reformers (Swedish Committee on the Funding and Organization of Health Services and Medical Care, 1993), the Dutch (Dutch Ministry of Welfare, Health and

Cultural Affairs, 1988), the Israelis (Israeli State Commission of Enquiry into the Israeli Health Care System, 1991) and, in the end, President Clinton (White House Domestic Policy Council, 1993) have all recommended that patients should have the choice of purchaser in their health reforms.

## Predictions

The preceding theory of contracting would lead us to predict that the scope for competitive efficiency gains would be least in the case of emergency services or life-threatening situations where the local hospital would tend to do a good job because of the professional satisfaction gained from life-saving work. The rewards from competition would be greatest in more repetitive non-emergency care, where a real choice of provider existed and where issues of patient convenience were important. These conditions, as it turns out, do coincide to a large extent with the boundaries of fundholders' hospital and community budgets.

On the other side of the balance sheet, more complex contracting with more providers done by multiple purchasers will be likely to be more expensive in administration, computing and professional time. The transaction costs will be high, to use the economic jargon. Small, isolated practices in the middle of a complex market, like inner London may find the costs of negotiation too great and their bargaining power low. We might postulate that both districts and GP fundholders will look for ways of minimizing their transaction costs, for example, by joint contracting, balancing them against the benefits they see in more complex contracting.

A different kind of efficiency gain will be reaped by enabling purchasers to switch services between hospital-based and practice-based care. Again, fundholding scores in theoretical terms compared with traditional budgeting, which puts bureaucratic budget boundaries around each of these activities.

Finally, purchasers will be influenced by the kind of information they have at their disposal and their capacity to analyse it. In this respect districts will have much more access to statistical material about district-based variations in patterns of disease and population characteristics. GPs will have professionally based judgements about quality, patients' complaints and preferences, as well as hospital prices and waiting times.

What, therefore, does theory suggest we might observe in the contracting arrangements made by fundholders and districts?

- Fundholders' contracts should give practices more capacity to exit and more choice than we should expect of districts, inhibited for the reasons we analysed earlier. We would expect GPs to be less tied to a single provider and to be seeking to create a contestable market, where at least one alternative provider could be used to play off against the other. Their capacity to do this will be affected by the local geography and hospital 'market'.
- We would expect fundholders to have gained more exacting quality requirements, especially as far as patient convenience and time were concerned.
- We would expect the contracts to be more flexible, with more case-by-case contracting, than districts.
- We would predict more switching between hospital inpatient, outpatient and practice-based care.
- We would expect fundholders to be less concerned with district-wide objectives and public health goals and to be more influenced by direct information about patient care, less by epidemiological information.

In what follows we examine the dynamics of purchasing in the practices and their associated districts to see how far these theoretical predictions hold.

## THE FIRST STEPS IN CONTRACTING

In 1991, not only was contracting new but the idea of GPs as purchasers of services was something with which hospitals found it very hard to come to terms. Most of the practices we interviewed in February 1991 had the same story to tell. Contract managers in most of the hospitals had not appreciated the implications of the scheme. They took the view that they would negotiate contracts with districts and GPs would simply accept them. Some thought fundholders so small an element that there was no reason to take any notice of them. A few trust and private hospitals were the only ones actively to seek fundholders' custom. Most of our sample had had no reply from their local hospitals to repeated requests to meet and discuss contracts in February 1991, two months before the scheme was to be operative. Several were still arguing and had not reached any contract by June, three months after the scheme had begun. By year two, and even more by year three, attitudes had changed remarkably. Hospitals had woken up to the fact that their survival depended on getting fundholders' money.

In 1991 hospitals expected GPs to make block contracts, specifying the same level of service with the same provider as the year before, just as districts were doing, and were told to do by the Government; 'keeping a steady state' it was called. None of our practices was prepared to do this.

'There is no point in us being in the scheme if that is all that happens' was the typical response. At the very least practices wanted to contract for only, perhaps, 80 per cent of their previous activity with a hospital, so that if the hospital did not perform as expected – took fewer patients, for example – the practice could switch part of its funds later in the year. It also gave the GPs some hold over the hospitals on quality. 'If we give them all our money at once they will ignore us.'

Right from the outset some practices began to make more complex contracts than the districts, using a mix of cost and volume, some block and some cost per case contracts. Cost and volume contracts gave the hospital an agreed volume of activity at a certain price. If more activity was purchased later it might be at a cheaper rate. Cost per case contracts went the whole way in flexibility. The hospital only got paid for the number of cases it actually did. This gave the practice the chance to send patients anywhere that would take them at any time. One of our practices went for all cost per case contracts in 1991 in the belief that this was the only way to keep the hospitals on their toes.

Most practices, however, did not want to break links with their established providers and set their main contracts with their traditional local provider. 'We want to make our local hospital the best.' But they also planned to diversify their suppliers and used the first year to test out alternatives on a small scale.

A summary of the first-wave contracts for our ten practices, as they were in April 1991, can be seen in Table 6.1. They contrasted with almost uniform block contracts, largely replicating existing provision, made by the districts.

The early contracting bore out other predictions we made earlier. Providers responded in ways that reflected their previous monopoly position. Their links with district staff proved very close. On the other hand, most of the practices wanted to change their use of at

**Table 6.1**    Contracts of first-wave practices, 1991–3

| Practice | Form of contract | |
|---|---|---|
| | *April 1991* | *April 1993* |
| 1 | Single block contract with DGH, except tests.<br>DHA contract specifications.<br>*Review:* undetermined, no formal contract agreed by June. | *Acute:* 1 main provider – cost per case – inpatients, cost and volume – outpatients, radiology – block; pathology – cost and volume, 4–5 other providers – cost per case. Mental health – block; physiotherapy – cost per case; community nursing – 1 provider – fixed price non-attributable contract.<br>*Quality specifications:* supplement DHA guidelines this year with own specifications.<br>*Review:* quarterly. |
| 2 | Cost and volume with two main providers. Some specialist cost per case contracts.<br>Quality specified by FHSA consortium of fundholders.<br>*Review:* monthly. | *Acute:* 1 main provider – cost and volume (marginal rates), other providers – cost per case, mental health, dietetics and chiropody – cost and volume, community nursing – 1 provider – fixed price non-attributable contract.<br>*Quality specifications:* detailed for acute, little change from DHA for community nursing.<br>*Review:* 3–6 months. |
| 3 | Seven different contracts with DGH, cost and volume, and block. Cost per case with two other local hospitals. Cost per case with two private hospitals.<br>Quality specified by practice.<br>*Review:* 6-monthly. | *Acute:* 1 main provider – cost per case in all areas; 5 other providers cost per case; community and mental health – cost per case; dietetics and chiropody – cost per case; community nursing (2 providers, but hope to contract with only 1) – fixed price non-attributable.<br>*Quality specifications:* detailed for acute, minor changes for community nursing.<br>*Review:* quarterly. |

**Table 6.1** Continued

| Practice | Form of contract | |
|---|---|---|
| | *April 1991* | *April 1993* |
| 4 | One provider – cost and volume. Practice's own quality specifications. Quality set by practice. *Review:* quarterly. | *Acute:* 2 main providers – cost and volume/cost per case hybrid (monthly payments, last two are adjusted according to activity); pathology and radiology – cost and volume, physiotherapy – cost per case, mental health – cost and volume, community nursing – 2 providers – fixed price non-attributable contracts. *Quality specifications:* Practice's own in conjunction with DHA, agreed with other local GPFH's little change to community nursing. *Review:* quarterly. |
| 5 | Two main providers – cost and volume; third similar, two others cost per case. Quality set by practice. *Review:* yearly. | *Acute:* 1 main provider; cost and volume for all areas apart from less used specialists, which will be cost per case; 4–5 other providers – cost per case; mental health, dietetics and chiropody – cost and volume; community nursing – 1 provider – fixed price non-attributable contracts. *Quality specifications:* as DHA, but practice has set own standards as well. This year it is to concentrate more on the quality of service at the point of access and discharge of patients. For community nursing it has set its own specifications (e.g. named staff in contract, strategies to enhance communications). *Review:* 6 months – acute, 3 months – community. |

**Table 6.1** Continued

| Practice | Form of contract | |
| --- | --- | --- |
| | *April 1991* | *April 1993* |
| 6 | Two main providers – cost per case; outpatient, physiotherapy and radiology – cost and volume. Quality set by consortium. *Review:* monthly. | *Acute:* 2 main providers – cost per case (with min. and max. volumes), 5 other providers – cost per case; mental health – cost per case; community nursing – 1 provider – fixed price non-attributable. *Quality specifications:* detailed agreed locally with other GPFH, community nursing – as DHA. *Review:* quarterly. |
| 7 | Main provider – cost and volume, pathology laboratory – block. Broad quality set as district. *Review:* yearly. | *Acute:* 1 main provider – all block contracts; 2 other providers – cost per case; community nursing – 2 providers – fixed price non-attributable; other community contracts – block. *Quality specifications:* as DHA specifications with practice supplements. *Review:* yearly. |
| 8 | Block contracts with DGH. Quality as district. *Review:* quarterly. | *Acute:* 1 main provider – cost per case (cost and zero volume) for all specialities including radiology; pathology – cost and volume; 5 other providers – cost per case; mental health – block; dietetics – block; chiropody – cost and volume; physiotherapy – cost and volume; community nursing – fixed price non-attributable. *Quality specifications:* as DHA, modified to include practice priorities; community nursing – little change although have specified that named nurses are provided. *Review:* 3-monthly. |

**Table 6.1** Continued

| Practice | Form of contract | |
|---|---|---|
| | *April 1991* | *April 1993* |
| 9 | Main provider block contract; cost per case second hospital. Quality as district but regular meetings with hospital on quality issues. *Review:* yearly. | *Acute:* 1 main provider – cost and volume (marginal rates above 80% activity), less used specialities – cost per case; radiology and pathology – fixed price non-attributable contract; 2 other providers – cost per case; mental health, dietetics and chiropody – cost and volume; community nursing – 1 provider – fixed price non-attributable contract. *Quality specifications:* as DHA, but with the addition of their own, agreed with other local GPFH, little change for community nursing. *Review:* 2-monthly. |
| 10 | One main provider – cost and volume. Separate pathology laboratory contract. Limited quality changes from district. Regular meetings with hospital. *Review:* yearly. | *Acute:* 2 main providers – 1 cost and volume and 1 cost per case; pathology and radiology – block; 2 other providers – cost and volume; community – mental health, chiropody and dietetics – block, community nursing – fixed price non-attributable. *Quality specifications:* as DHA in conjunction with practice's priorities. *Review:* 3–6-monthly. |

least one speciality in the first year because of dissatisfaction with the service. The hospitals' response was often very hostile. One phoned the practice manager to demand what she thought she was doing? 'It's our money you have taken. You have no right to take it elsewhere.'

When practices tried to include quality specifications, for example, about the speed with which the GP received discharge letters, the response was very negative, districts were not asking for such things and everyone would be treated alike. When the hospitals' contract managers did agree to such items the consultants objected. One contract had been agreed in good time but in April, after the contract should have begun the consultants finally saw it and woke up. They raised objections. One meeting, called for consultants to confront the GPs who, as a group controlled a significant part of the hospital's budget, ended in disarray. The consultants blamed the managers for making such contracts; the fundholders looked on amused. One of them said, 'It's all about your power. You can't bear the thought you are not top dogs any more. That's what it's all about.'

Mostly, however, diplomacy and the long view prevailed. One group of fundholders was aware that it would be pointless to impose a set of unattainable quality targets. It went instead for regular meetings with the local managers and consultants to discuss ways of improving standards and to take up general issues of concern. In June 1991, after a couple of reminders and delays the first meeting took place. One of the doctors present said afterwards, 'I realized that this was a historical event. For the first time ever we had managed to get to talk to the consultants about the standard of care they were giving our patients.'

Most practices were also very sensitive to the charge that they were getting something that would not be available to patients of non-fundholders, and often insisted that anything they negotiated should be available to other GPs.

Every one of our practices had been unhappy with their pathology testing service. Most practices had to wait a week for the return of their specimens. Often the information was poorly presented. Tests for the same patient would arrive on different days and have to be matched. In every case, bar two, the practices were able to improve their services quite dramatically. Most gained daily delivery and improved information. Once the laboratory agreed to provide this level of service for fundholders it had to accept it was possible for non-fundholders too. The stories told by the practices were very similar. In most cases responses from the hospital that no alteration to service was feasible changed when the practice quoted much better arrangements that had been offered by another hospital or a private laboratory. In other cases the practices did change supplier, two to a private firm.

This experience illustrates some of the theoretical points made earlier. Routine laboratory testing is a boring and not very rewarding job. There is no direct patient contact. GPs are remote from the laboratory. Whereas hospital consultants can phone up and complain to a colleague, there is nothing much a GP can do if he or she does not get a test on time. There is plenty of scope for X-inefficiency to creep in. There is also a real contestable market once GPs have the power to spend their own money. As one fundholder demonstrated, it is possible for a laboratory several hundred miles away to supply results overnight. Every practice had several possible alternative suppliers to choose from. Given a real market challenge to an established monopoly the quality of service improved.

Other initial changes were less dramatic but still significant. One practice had for years had complaints from its women patients about one consultant. Attempts to move to a more distant hospital had failed – there was no reason for this hospital to increase its already high workload. Now it had money to pay, the practice offered to switch all its patients. The consultant agreed to take them; he was able to fund a new post as a result.

In another case, a practice switched gynaecology from the local hospital which was good but had a two-year waiting list; it did the same with its orthopaedics and ophthalmology. The new hospital was 20 miles away but the waiting list was less than six months. Again, nearly all the patients were pleased with the change. The few who were not were offered the option of going to the local hospital with a longer wait.

In another case the local dermatology department had a long waiting time; people with skin conditions could wait up to nine months and there was no difference in waiting time between serious and non-serious cases. The partners knew a local specialist who now acted privately. She agreed to take less serious cases and guarantee to see them within two weeks. She offered a below-private-rate consultancy fee for this monthly contract. This worked so well that it was made a regular part of the practice's service.

Some practices were keen for consultants to visit to do outpatient clinics. One GP explained there were always a lot of patients whom he could not help but who needed 'the white coat treatment' – the final authority that this was the case. Yet there was a long wait and a difficult journey to the county hospital. This was discussed at one of the regular meetings with consultants and it was agreed that a monthly or bimonthly clinic could deal with all these cases and, if any were serious and merited a full outpatient referral, this could be arranged. The consultant got through more cases than normal and was prepared to charge less per referral. One practice transferred all outpatient work to its surgery.

The fact that GPs were now paying for outpatient visits also made them consider their value. GPs complained of 'the Senior House Officer syndrome'. A junior doctor saw a patient in an outpatient clinic and tended to play safe and say, 'Come back in six months' knowing that he or she would not be there. GPs felt they could often do a better monitoring job anyway. Now they wrote into their contracts a limit to the number of repeat visits without their approval.

These were small but important changes designed to improve the quality of the service their patients were receiving by reducing hospital inefficiency.

A second group of innovations concerned services of a simple nature, which could be offered in the practice and which both speeded access and relieved pressure on the GP. An example was counselling. Many doctors were critical of the psychiatric outpatient service, which was often the only referral a GP felt they could make for a mildly depressed individual or someone suffering from marriage problems or bereavement. There was a general view that this was a waste of time or worse. A better use of their budget was to employ a counsellor. A number already did so on a limited scale financed out of the partnership income. Fundholding offered greater scope. Others argued that they hoped to save money on their anti-inflammatory drug costs by employing a physiotherapist.

A different kind of example was afforded by one practice that used its patients' questionnaire to ask not only about the practice's services but about the hospital. What did patients most want to see improved? Car parking facilities was the reply. This was included in the contract discussions with the hospital and a promise to extend the car park was obtained.

In short, the practices in 1991 did use their bargaining power to some effect. The extent to which they were able to do so varied. Our smallest practice in the middle of the complex London market, for example, found it difficult to get much leverage.


## A FAIR ACCOUNT?

When we gave an account of this more active and effective purchasing in our interim report (Glennerster, Matsaganis and Owens,

1992) various objections were raised at seminars and conferences. One was that our comparison with districts was unfair. Districts had had their hands tied by Government; this was the reason they had been less innovative. Another criticism was that what we were observing was confined to an unrepresentative group of exceptional first-wavers. A third objection was that it was only because so few practices were in the scheme that they were getting exceptional treatment. It would be impossible to sustain when more practices joined. Objections of a different kind came from harder evidence. In the Oxford Region, Bradlow and Coulter (1993) suggested that there had been no significant changes in referrals by fundholders. Fundholding was making no difference. Now, with two more years experience and third-wave practices in our sample, we can consider the validity of these objections.

The inescapable conclusion, we believe, is that the later rounds of contracting reinforce the conclusions we reached in our preliminary report.

**More demanding and diverse contracts by first-wavers**

Despite the removal of the ministerial constraint on setting new contracts, districts have been slow to develop innovative or aggressive contracting. Purchasing has tended to be provider-driven. Districts have been very concerned to stabilize the market and protect their existing hospitals (though not those in central London). As one district contracts manager explained:

> We really are committed to setting block contracts. Providers are relying on our money. We can't withhold money in the same way as fundholders can. However, we are making moves towards setting cost and volume contracts in some areas. Things are changing.

The DoH's planning guidance for 1994–5, in fact, required districts to move away from simple block contracts. The quality specifications set by districts focused on the statutory Patient's Charter standards (Department of Health, 1991). They primarily reflected central political objectives with some supplementary regional and local additions. They tended to be general statements of the service quality the authorities would like to see providers achieve. To be more detailed or idiosyncratic was simply too costly in administrative time and they felt they would never be able to monitor such contracts.

In contrast, as we can see from Table 6.1, our fundholders developed the complexity and range of their contracts beyond those of the first year. They were more likely to be set out in a way that enabled the GPs to measure performance against targets. Only one practice had kept to a block contract with their main provider. Most had gone for cost and volume contracts, some of a rather sophisticated kind. The more cases the practice put with the hospital at the end of the year the cheaper the price on a sliding scale. In another case the volumes were reassessed every month. There had been an increase in the number of cost per case contracts despite the administrative burdens. The computer record systems and the prompter billing from the hospitals now made cost per case contracts more feasible. It gave the hospitals more direct incentive to keep up a regular flow of work. One practice had switched all its out-patient cost per case arrangements to a payment per completed episode rather than per referral – 'It worked like a dream.'

The hospitals were also coming up with much more flexible deals than the first-wavers had been offered with high discount rates, up to 50 per cent off, for cases beyond the agreed volume, with special rates for particular specialities. One gave block contracts for all the pathology work but, if the volume was not met the surplus could be used in the rest of the hospital. The second development we noted was the diversification of providers the practices were using. The first-wavers were now less dependent on a single local main provider (see Table 6.1). All had begun to use a range of other providers. Our original predictions had been sustained.

What of our critics' objections?

## Third-wavers go further

It was certainly plausible to argue that all we were seeing in our first-wave practices in 1991 was a quite exceptional group of able and enthusiastic doctors who would in no way be indicators of things to come. This has not proved the case. Of course, our third-wavers may be exceptional too, but what is interesting is that, as a group, they have learned from the experience of the first-wavers in contracting and taken off from there. The sophistication of the contracts themselves and the use of alternative providers was greater in the case of the third-wavers.

In the third wave, eight out of the 16 practices had begun by deliberately making contracts with two main providers (Table 6.2).

**Table 6.2** Third-wave contracting

| Practice | |
|---|---|
| 11 | *Form of contract:* acute – 1 main provider – cost and volume, radiology and pathology – block; 5–6 other providers – cost per case; mental health and other community – cost and volume; community nursing – 1 provider – fixed price non-attributable contracts.<br>*Quality specifications:* as DHA, with a few additions from the practice, community nursing – unchanged.<br>*Review:* quarterly. |
| 12 | *Form of contract:* acute – 2 main providers – cost per case; pathology and radiology – cost and volume; 4–5 other providers – cost per case; community, mental health, chiropody and dietetics – cost and volume, community nursing – 2 providers – fixed price non-attributable.<br>*Quality specifications:* as DHA, modified to include practice priorities, detailed community.<br>*Review:* quarterly. |
| 13 | *Form of contract:* acute – 2 main providers – 1 cost and volume (with marginal rates), the other cost per case; radiology and pathology – block; 3 other providers – cost per case; mental health and other community contracts – block; community nursing – 1 provider – fixed price non-attributable contract.<br>*Quality specifications:* as DHA, with practice supplement for acute and community nursing.<br>*Review:* monthly to begin with and then quarterly. |
| 14 | *Form of contract:* acute – 1 main provider – cost per case; radiology and pathology – block; 3–4 other providers – cost per case; mental health and other community – block; community nursing – 1 provider – fixed price non-attributable contract.<br>*Quality specifications:* as DHA, with supplement from the practice agreed locally with other GPFH.<br>*Review:* quarterly. |
| 15 | *Form of contract:* acute – 1 main provider – all cost per case; 4 other providers – all cost per case; mental health and other community contracts – block; community nursing – 1 provider – fixed price non-attributable contract.<br>*Quality specifications:* as DHA with practice supplement as agreed with other local GPFH.<br>*Review:* quarterly. |
| 16 | *Form of contract:* acute – 1 main provider – cost and zero volume; radiology and pathology – block; 2 other providers – cost and volume; mental health – block; chiropody and dietetics – cost per case, community nursing – 1 provider – fixed price non-attributable contract.<br>*Quality specifications:* detailed – seen as 'targets' to work towards agreed with local GPFH group.<br>*Review:* quarterly. |

**Table 6.2**    Continued

| Practice |
| --- |

17      *Form of contract:* acute – 2 main providers – cost and volume (with marginal rates); pathology and radiology – block; 3 other providers – cost per case; mental health – block; community nursing – 1 provider – fixed price non-attributable contracts.
*Quality specifications:* as DHA with practice supplement for acute; little changed for community nursing.
*Review:* 3-monthly.

18      *Form of contract:* acute – 1 main provider – cost per case (with discounts for marginal costs); pathology and radiology – cost and volume; 5 other providers – cost per case; mental health – block; community nursing – 2 providers – fixed price non-attributable contracts.
*Quality specifications:* detailed, community nursing as DHA with practice supplement.
*Review:* monthly, contracts renewed 6-monthly.

19      *Form of contract:* acute – 2 main providers – all cost per case; pathology and radiology – block; small contracts with 2 other providers – cost per case; mental health – block; chiropody and dietetics – block; community nursing – 2 providers – fixed price non-attributable contracts.
*Quality specifications:* expanded upon DHA guidelines, put more emphasis on some issues; community nursing – detailed.
*Review:* quarterly.

20      *Form of contract:* acute – 1 main provider – cost and volume (above 75% activity – marginal costs); radiology – block; pathology – in negotiation; 3 other providers – cost per case but offered one-off special deals on small volumes; community – all block, community nursing – 1 provider – fixed price non-attributable.

21      *Form of contract:* acute – 1 main provider – cost and zero volume; pathology and radiology – block; 10 other providers – cost per case; community – block; community nursing – 1 provider – fixed price non-attributable contracts.
*Quality specifications:* detailed, supplement to DHA, agreed with other local GPFH; community nursing – detailed supplement.
*Review:* quarterly.

22      *Form of contract:* acute – 2 main providers – cost per case (although sensitive to volume to gain marginal costs); pathology and radiology – block; 2 other providers – cost per case; mental health – cost and volume; other community contracts – block; community nursing – 1 provider (previously 3) – fixed price non-attributable contract.
*Quality specifications:* acute and community – as DHA with minor additions.
*Review:* 3-monthly.

**Table 6.2** Continued

---

*Practice*

---

23    *Form of contract:* acute – 1 main provider – cost and volume; pathology
      and radiology – block; 3 other providers – cost per case; community –
      block; community nursing – fixed price non-attributable contracts.
      *Quality specifications:* as DHA, supplements agreed by local GPFH;
      community nursing – unchanged.
      *Review:* quarterly.

24    *Form of contract:* acute – 2 main providers – cost per case (zero
      volume); radiology and pathology – block; 2 other providers – cost per
      case; mental health and other community contracts – block; community
      nursing – 1 provider – fixed price non-attributable contracts.
      *Quality specifications:* as DHA, with minor additions, no change to
      community nursing.
      *Review:* quarterly.

25    *Form of contract:* acute – 2 main providers – cost and volume (marginal
      rates); outpatient reattendance – block; pathology – block; 3 other
      providers – cost per case; mental health and other community contracts
      – cost and volume; community nursing – 2 providers – fixed price
      non-attributable contracts.
      *Quality specifications:* detailed for acute agreed with local GPFH,
      minor changes for community nurses.
      *Review:* quarterly.

26    *Form of contract:* acute – 2 main providers: (i) cost and volume (ii) cost
      per case – inpatients, cost and volume – outpatients; pathology and
      radiology – block; mental health – block; chiropody and dietetics –
      block; community nursing – 2 providers – fixed price non-attributable
      contracts.
      *Quality specifications:* acute – adopting local GP fundholders' group
      standardized contract with minor additions by the practice; community
      nursing – as DHA.
      *Review:* quarterly.

---

This often formalized existing relations with more than one acute
provider but the practices moved to more equal sharing to keep
each provider on their toes. What was it the practices were looking
for?

**Responsiveness**

Two practices, far apart geographically, had almost identical stories
to tell. Though good, the regional teaching hospital consultants had
poor reputations as far as responsive service was concerned –

**Table 6.3**   GP contracts: examples of specifications

---

*1) Information required from providers*
Most practices set out in their contracts information requirements that they wanted supplied by providers. This was seen to be important to assess performance of providers and aid activity and financial monitoring for practices.

Outpatients:
On a monthly basis:
  (a)   number of first visits for assessment and for treatment by speciality and referring GP;
  (b)   total number of assessments, attendances.
On a quarterly basis:
  (a)   number of letters of referral by speciality and GP;
  (b)   number of DNAs and cancellations by speciality;
  (c)   results of medical audit.
Annually:
  (a)   results of consumer surveys;
  (b)   results of sample surveys to review waiting times and reasons for waiting, period between receipt of GP letter of referral and first appointment.

Inpatients:
On a monthly basis:
  (a)   number of inpatient and day case elective episodes completed by speciality, procedure and average length of stay;
  (b)   number of patients admitted to a waiting list with admission dates given by speciality.
Quarterly:
  (a)   number of practice patients on waiting list by length of time waiting and by speciality;
  (b)   number of postoperative infections and number of readmissions by speciality.
Annually:
  (a)   results of consumer surveys;
  (b)   results of surveys to review waiting times:
      – between date decision to admit and actual date of admission;
      – between arrival at the hospital and accommodation in a bed.

Community nursing:
Monthly:
  (a)   number and type of contracts and treatment performed by HVs and DNs by new referrals and follow-ups;
  (b)   overall time spent on the above contracts and treatment, travelling and administrative duties by individual HVs and DNs;
  (c)   all referrals made by the community nurses within the scope of the scheme.
Quarterly:
  (a)   provide caseload analysis and community health profiles to the practice;
  (b)   overall cost to the provider of HVs and DNs allotted to the practice;
  (c)   overall overhead costs to the practice allotted to the practice by expenditure headings.

---

**Table 6.3** Continued

---

*2) Communication with GPs*

One problem that irritated most practices was the poor communication that they had with individual consultants. It was frequently felt that they were not kept adequately informed about their patient's condition or progress, and in some cases discharge letters were scrappy or else did not arrive until weeks after they left hospital. Practices were therefore keen to improve the quality and speed of communication. For example:

'. . . provider will inform the patient's GP of results of assessments within 5 working days of the last assessment attendance.'

'. . . provider will inform patient's GP at the earliest opportunity if very difficult clinical problems occur.'

'. . . inform GP within 5 working days of patient's formal discharge from hospital.'

'. . . comprehensive and legible discharge summary to be sent within 2 weeks, but letter immediately on discharge with full explanation of drugs, procedures, management and findings.'

*3) Courtesy to patients*

Although DHA contracts did include aspects relating to providers' courtesy to patients, GPFH contracts were again more specific and asked for better standards to be worked towards. For example:

'Notify the patient of receipt of the letter of referral indicating how long he/she will have to wait for an appointment within 5 working days.'

'The patient will be given a minimum of 2 weeks notice before admission.'

'24 hours notice must be given to a relative/carer before discharge.'

'The patient must not wait longer than 2 hours before being accommodated in a bed.'

*4) Waiting times*

Fundholding contracts were more likely to set out shorter waiting times for providers to work towards. Furthermore, most wanted providers to give them information, when possible, on their performance. For example:

'Patient should wait no longer than 6 weeks from time of referral to appointment and only one week in urgent cases.'

'In outpatients . . . 90% of patients should wait no longer than 30 minutes and 100% no longer than 60 minutes.'

'Life threatening conditions should be admitted for investigation within 3 weeks of outpatient appointment.'

'If an operation is cancelled, the patient must be offered another date within 4 weeks of cancellation.'

'. . . if the first appointment is likely to exceed 8 weeks waiting time, the provider is required to notify the purchaser so that suitable arrangements can be made with another provider.'

---

'classic prima donnas', 'simply not interested in speeding up or doing routine work', 'if the waiting list is too long take your patients elsewhere, seems to be their attitude'. So the doctors did go elsewhere. There was a small hospital where the consultants were keen for work, very keen to reduce waiting times, worked well with the managers and were eager to respond to the GPs' suggestions. Both practices had decided to transfer their custom steadily, testing how things went, even though in one case this meant about a 20-mile journey. Waiting times and responsiveness were all-important. In another case where two providers were almost equidistant, the practice said they would divide the contract in the first year and see which responded best.

### Supporting a local service

Most said they wanted to use their local provider or the provider they had traditionally used. They wanted to protect a local service that could be there in an emergency, but they also wanted to improve it. They often took a stronger line on this than their districts. 'It is not in our interests to run it down.' 'They provide a good service. I am not going to change to save a small amount of money.' Others felt it their responsibility to give financial stability to the local provider, in one case a new trust.

The extreme example of local support was mentioned in Chapter 5, where a group of local practices had joined fundholding precisely to save the local hospital. In our last interview with them they were delighted that the local community unit was to take the hospital on, using it partly for their purposes but also running hospital facilities, kept going in large part by the assured referrals of local fundholding GPs. Without their money the scheme would not have been viable. Their patients' views about inconvenience had weighed heavily with them.

### Detailed quality specifications

Over the three years the practices had come to evolve a more demanding set of additional specifications than the districts, of which we give examples in Table 6.3. By the third wave there were more groups of GPs wanting to agree common quality specifications. They recognized that if every fundholder went for a different set they would have no chance of being met.

### Preference for the NHS

In nearly all cases there was a strong preference for contracts with an NHS provider. All had been approached by the private sector but wanted NHS money to stay in the NHS. Only where they had particular problems would they contemplate private contracting.

## The larger the market share the larger the impact

It had been plausible to suggest that we might merely be seeing exceptional treatment of a few practices in the first wave. They might be being offered special deals at marginal cost while the bulk of services were offered to districts at lower quality. All this would go when fundholding spread. Again, the very reverse seems to be the case. Amongst our first-wave practices, those who have gained least are those who have been isolated fundholders, only one in an area of non-fundholders. Those who have had most impact on the providers have been those in areas where over half or, in one case, nearly all practices went fundholding. The same has been true of third-wavers. The hospitals in the county where nearly two-thirds of the population are in fundholding practices have been shaken, and indeed the very structure of the service has been transformed by the sheer market power of the fundholders.

## Fundholders force change

'To be frank we should have pulled the plug ourselves years ago' one manager said. 'But our hands were tied. We've just been propping them up.' In one district an official encouraged an influential practice to go for fundholding in order to give the district leverage over a particularly intransigent group of consultants in a local hospital. He knew he stood no hope of getting the district to withdraw the whole contract from this team – all the other consultants would have rallied round. Fundholding GPs were independent and flexible enough to exercise their power of exit.

In another area where most of the GPs had become fundholders the community trust changed its internal organization in order to respond. It knew its very existence depended on keeping the GPs' custom and agreed to negotiate packages of service tailored to each practice. It wanted to preserve certain common standards, training and approaches, but accepted the case would have to be won by argument. The whole, more responsive organizational structure had been produced by the existence of a large block of fundholders.

In the areas where very few fundholders existed the impact on the community services had been negligible.

**Referral patterns**

Table 6.4 summarizes the changes in referrals in our first-wave practices where comparable statistics could be extracted.

Though economists talk easily about exercising the sanction of exit and draw analogies with customers going to another shop, GPs do not think like that. The dilemma Hirschman (1970) discusses was very evident. Loyalty, professional and personal links, and sympathy for the difficulties their hospital colleagues face, make them reluctant to act. One group talked rather ferociously about changing providers in London, but in the end changed very little, reluctant to upset relations more than necessary. One of our first-wave practices had expressed dissatisfaction with the service they received from a famous local teaching hospital in our very first interview back in 1990. By early 1993 they were still sending most of their patients there. The new part-time fundholding manager, retired from a large national retailer, suggested they should begin to move their contracts. The partners went through great heart searching. We arrived to interview them shortly afterwards and the difficulty of the decision was plain. 'I didn't understand the attitude', the manager said. 'It is a different mentality. But in the end they agreed. They had waited three years for things to change.'

The third-wavers were less inhibited than the first-wavers had been. As we mentioned in Chapter 5, one practice had not been happy with the psychiatric service they had been receiving for many years. The lead fundholding GP said:

> The consultants don't know what is happening in the community and don't want to know either. They provide a very poor service. We took a decision (not to contract with them but to go to a neighbouring area for the whole service, acute as well, with a special dispensation). They took it very badly, but we stuck to our guns.

At a later interview he said:

> We are delighted with the service we are now getting. We can refer to a named consultant, we have clinics at the practice and communication has improved tremendously. For the first time

**Table 6.4**   Changes in referrals by first-wave practices (percentage referrals)

|  | Prefundholding (1990) | Postfundholding (1993) |
| --- | --- | --- |
| *Practice A* | | |
| Hospital 1 | 85 | 50 |
| Hospital 2 | 10 | 38 |
| Other NHS | 5 | 5 |
| Private | – | 5 |
| Inhouse | – | 2 |

Waiting times reduced in orthopaedics, gynaecology and ophthalmology (42–21 weeks) by providers responding to competition and by moving gynaecology. Referral rates up 8%.

|  | | |
| --- | --- | --- |
| *Practice B* | | |
| Hospital 1 | 90 | 60 |
| Hospital 2 | 5 | 5 |
| Other NHS | 5 | 25 |
| Private | – | 5 |
| Inhouse | – | 5 |

Ophthalmology improved in time and responsiveness by switching. Referrals overall about the same level.

|  | | |
| --- | --- | --- |
| *Practice C* | | |
| Hospital 1 | 99 | 85 |
| Hospital 2 | – | 6 |
| Hospital 3 | – | 4 |
| Other NHS | 1 | – |
| Inhouse and private | – | 5 |

|  | | |
| --- | --- | --- |
| *Practice D* | | |
| Hospital 1 | 95 | 80 |
| Hospital 2 | 5 | 2 |
| Hospital 3 | – | 5 |
| Hospital 4 | – | 5 |
| Hospital 5 | – | 5 |
| Inhouse | – | – |
| Private | – | 3 |

Referrals down a little.

**Table 6.4**   Continued

|  | Prefundholding (1990) | Postfundholding (1993) |
|---|---|---|
| *Practice E* | | |
| Hospital 1 | 48 | 7 |
| Hospital 2 | 48 | 75 |
| Other NHS | 4 | 3 |
| Inhouse | – | 10 |
| Private | – | 5 |
| *Practice F* | | |
| Hospital 1 | 98 | 99 |
| Other NHS | 2 | 1 |
| Inhouse | – | – |
| Private | – | – |

Activity was 39% up in 1991–2 over 1990 and 17.5% up in 1992–3 on previous year despite making savings. Major improvement in provider efficiency.

we know what is happening to our patients. I have heard things have changed with the first team. They were leant on when they lost our contract.

The message did not seem to have got through to all pathology departments either. One third-wave practice produced an account very reminiscent of our first-wave interviews. They had got a very negative response to requests for a collection service and a quicker turn around. They investigated a range of alternatives and found a private firm offering all they wanted at a competitive price and also the services of a phlebotomist. The hospital responded belatedly. Now all GPs in the area have a collection service *and* a phlebotomist.

In other cases our third-wavers had improved matters by merely threatening to move. One practice was very unhappy about the dermatology service and had been pressing for changes for a long time to no avail. Patients had to wait nine to ten months to get an appointment. 'Both consultants have a flourishing private practice but are providing a shoddy NHS service. They won't listen to anybody.' The practice began exploring the services of a consultant from a distant hospital to come in and see patients. 'The managers got wind of this and leant on the consultants. We got a promise that things would improve.'

In another case a practice in a small market town was unhappy with a consultant who visited the local cottage hospital. He was supposed to hold weekly clinics there. He rarely turned up, often for weeks on end. They and the other fundholding practices in the town told the hospital they had had enough. The hospital was not surprised at the complaint but it gave them (the managers) the opportunity to get him to go. He was given early retirement.

## Community services

These contracts were difficult to judge because the first-year contracting was hedged around with much stricter rules. Fundholders had to make contracts with NHS units or trusts. The contracts had to be fixed-price non-attributable block contracts. The practices hoped and expected that the constraints would be temporary and were upset when the DoH continued the restrictions into 1994–5. Their initial view was that they were simply being asked to hand back a block of money to community services and that the whole thing was a charade.

The community units were responsible for setting a price based on what had happened in the past year and allocating management costs pro rata. Most providers were very secretive about how they were actually calculating the costs. 'They seem to have pulled the figures out of the air and are not prepared to explain or discuss them.'

What made things so frustrating for the practices was that they had little or no information of their own about what services their patients were receiving from the community services. No doubt this reflected past disinterest, but now they were supposed to be paying, the practices wanted to know which patients were receiving such services as chiropody, dietetics and mental health support. In about half the cases the community units refused to tell the practices and instructed their nurses and heath visitors not to tell the practices anything. A number of our GPs said they would seek to go to providers outside their areas if the community services did not co-operate. 'If we are buying a service it is only right we should know what we are getting.' Some of the nurses thought the GPs ought to know and agreed to share their diaries with the practices. Most community units began by being hostile to the changes and were determined to treat the fundholders in a 'take it or leave it mode', just as the hospital providers had three years before. By the time of our summer 1993 interviews attitudes had begun to change. The units responded to the fact that the number of fundholders was rising fast. We quoted earlier the example of one trust that had changed its stance and marketed its services right from the outset, and this approach was being followed by more community units.

Most GPs wanted staff based at the practice. Few wanted to be able to employ the community staff directly but most GPs wanted to be on the appointing panels for staff they were to work with. They wanted to extend the role of community nurses to include domiciliary electrocardiograms (ECGs) and blood taking, catheterization and immunizations. These were things nurses could do.

Most wanted to integrate community nurses with practice nurses' work. They felt the services were managerially top heavy and too expensive. 'We could double the number of staff if we did it ourselves', was one view.

One region decided that the information on budget setting was so poor it would simply allocate a nominal budget to the activity, pay the practice that and then require the practice to pay it back – 'Totally pointless exercise.'

In several cases the community services had quoted very low prices. The tactics were fairly clear. A very low quote would lead to a very low budget. This would then become the norm and the practice would not then be able to shift its custom elsewhere to a provider that was charging realistic prices. Only a *per capita* formula-based budget would prevent such provider capture tactics.

The practices felt, by the summer of 1993, that they had, at least, begun a dialogue with their community service colleagues and begun to understand better what they were doing.

## CONCLUSION: CONTESTABLE MARKETS EXIST

We can now return to the propositions we made at the outset of this chapter. Most of those predictions have, in our view, been borne out – in those services covered by fundholding, GPs have been better contractors than their districts. Fundholding practices did act on their own detailed experience of hospital services and patient views about the way they were treated and convenience issues. The practices were more prepared to use the power of exit to improve the quality of the hospital services they received. Even in rural areas the range of non-emergency procedures covered in the fundholding list can be contracted relatively easily with hospitals 20 or 30 miles away. Patients have been willing and happy to travel further, if it reduced their waiting time appreciably. Practices have been prepared to arrange and pay for transport where necessary. In more metropolitan areas a range of services exist much nearer at hand. One of our suburban practices did a complete trawl of feasible market options and concluded they had 60 providers available.

## Breaking boundaries

Practices did begin to challenge the traditional boundary lines between hospital and primary care and between community and primary care. During the three years, what one of our practices called 'a sea change' occurred in consultants' willingness to come out to practices to do clinics, screen patients and pick out cases needing more facilities or treatment. Consultants came to appreciate that the practices' appointment systems worked more effectively than the hospitals'; the support staff were usually better. Patients turned up, knowing the receptionist would give reminders and communicate displeasure at non-attendance, whereas hospital outpatients had a large absence rate. Patients knew the surgery and tended to be more relaxed. There were practical limits, however. Consultants could not spend all their time out in surgeries, their junior staff needed to be trained by participating in the outpatient work. Hospital managers became concerned about the drain on the hospital availability of consultant staff. Fundholders had a response to this. In the third round of contracting groups of fundholders were combining to offer clinic facilities in a small town and clinicians were coming with their junior staff who enjoyed the chance to get out of the hospital. The growth of fundholding was providing the opportunity to change the boundaries of care. None of this was, of course, impossible under old health service arrangements. There was, however, no incentive for them to happen. What the edge of competition has done is to provide that catalyst.

If GPs *are* better at contracting non-emergency treatment, and perhaps other treatment too, this raises the issue of equity. Why should these advantages be denied to the patients of most GPs?

## The costs

The other side to this story is that it is more costly in administration. The transaction costs are higher. Each practice is negotiating its own needs with the hospitals. This takes the time of a senior partner and the practice manager or a contracts manager. The computer system has to keep account of referrals and of bills paid. A management allowance is given to practices. The hospitals and community services had to gear themselves to negotiate with practices. This often meant a dedicated fundholding contracts manager and contact person. The FHSA had to have a separate fundholding capacity, to set the budgets, oversee spending and advise new fundholders. Regions needed a fundholding officer, part of their finance staff had to be assigned to produce a budget-setting methodology, track the budgets and keep them down so far as possible. The DoH has been running various pilot schemes to see if it is possible to reduce the administrative costs and to reap some economies of scale in administration.

One of our regions attempted a costing exercise to see what the total administrative costs of the system were. They included all the management allowances, extra equipment costs and the costs of FHSA and regional staff. They also included the costs of the preliminary year allowance, which might not be appropriate for a steady-state calculation. On the other hand, they did not attempt to cost the time and resources devoted by hospitals to GPs' billing. They concluded that the costs amounted to an additional 2 per cent of the revenue expenditure concerned.

The question is, therefore, is the GP fundholding system of contracting worth the extra cost?

In posing this question it is important to recognize that the extra administrative expenditure also brings spin-off benefits. First, the individualized information fundholders and hospitals needed to generate was useful in itself. Hospitals had to improve their patient data and discharge systems, informing GPs more promptly. All this improved the clinical quality and continuity of the care patients received. The second kind of gain has been the benefits of improved management for the whole practice that has flown from being able to employ a really good manager as opposed to a senior clerk to run the practice.

We assess the balance sheet in Chapter 12.

# 7

# CONTAINING THE DRUGS BUDGET

While a major purpose behind the fundholding scheme was to increase the efficiency of hospitals and community services, a second and less publicized purpose was to contain GPs' own pre-scribing costs. Pharmaceutical expenditure has been one of the fastest-growing elements in the NHS budget. If we are to under-stand this part of the fundholding scheme we need to see it in the context of these longer-term attempts to contain drugs spending and the economics of pharmaceutical spending.

## THE ECONOMICS OF PHARMACEUTICALS

Unlike other NHS services, the production of pharmaceuticals has always been undertaken by the private market for profit. The NHS has merely purchased the industry's products. There has always been a purchaser–provider split, although the extent of competition has been restricted. In order to survive, a pharmaceutical company must be continually inventing and marketing new drugs; it has to invest a lot in research and development. Pharmaceuticals is one of the few British industries to have done this successfully. Once a new drug is invented and tested and the results are available in the medical journals, knowledge about how to make it becomes poten-tially available to all the company's rivals, who could then produce it cheaply, free-riding on the expensive research and development costs of the original company. To prevent this, competition is limited for a period after the invention of the drug under patent. No other company can copy the drug and produce it until the patent expires. But who are the purchasers? In the United Kingdom there

are three main kinds of purchaser: the ordinary individual consumer who buys medicines over the counter in the chemist's shop,
NHS hospitals and GPs who prescribe for their patients. Patients
may have to pay a prescription charge at the chemist in this last case
but about 85 per cent of those who get prescriptions are exempt
from paying because they are elderly or poor or have a chronic
condition.

Roughly speaking, the private consumer pays for one-fifth of the
total expenditure on drugs in the United Kingdom. Another fifth is
purchased by NHS hospitals but three-fifths derives from the
demand generated by GPs prescribing for their patients.

Without any Government interference in this process GPs would
have an open chequebook – the Government agreeing to pay
whatever they recommend to their patients. In economic terms the
system would resemble a system where third-party health insurers
are forced to pay bills generated by demanders who have no budget
constraint.

The pharmaceutical industry went through a revolution in the
1950s and 1960s. Until the 1930s only 100 or so drug patents were
issued a year and even in 1945 it was no more than about 500. By the
mid-1960s new patents were running at over 6000 a year. Drug
company advertising grew in scale and sophistication, pushing at
the GPs' open chequebook.

Between 1978 and 1988 the real-terms growth in drug spending
was 5 per cent per annum, at a time when overall NHS hospital
spending had been constrained to 1 or 2 per cent, or even less in
some years. GPs' share of total drugs expenditure also rose in the
same period. The Treasury's concern to get this aspect of NHS
spending under control was understandable.

## PAST ATTEMPTS TO HOLD THE LINE

Treasury concern, indeed, dates back to the passing of the 1911
National Insurance Act, which first enabled GPs to prescribe at
public expense. From the outset the Government tried to control
panel doctors' prescribing. A cash-limited Drug Fund was created,
which was meant to set a limit to what panel doctors could prescribe. A panel doctor who strayed too far from the local average
was likely to receive a visit from the Regional Medical Officer
(Martin, 1957).

In 1948 the cash-limited Drug Fund was abolished and expenditure on drugs was deemed to be 'demand-led', or based on GPs' determination of need. Public expenditure would follow demand. This happy notion was soon seen to be incompatible with economy in public spending and in 1954 a Standing Committee on the Classification of Proprietary Preparations was set up to 'advise' on what drugs GPs should prescribe. They could go beyond it but would have to justify doing so. GPs could only prescribe 'expensive' drugs if a price had been agreed with the pharmaceutical industry. What the Government began to do was to use its potential monopsony power to bargain down prices in the sector. This led to a voluntary profit-limiting scheme between the industry and Government.

This mix of dual pressure both on the GP and the industry remained the basis of cost containment for the next three decades, though the sophistication of the methods grew and committees came and went (Martin, 1957; Sainsbury Committee, 1967; Reekie and Weber, 1979).

It was the coming of the Conservative Government in 1979 that prompted a change of approach. The first move was to impose a limited 'selected list' of therapeutic categories, limiting Exchequer reimbursement in 'non-essential' categories. This had some effect, reducing the drugs bill by £75 million, according to the Government (Department of Health, 1989a). In addition the Government tried the voluntary approach. It improved the information each practice received about the cost of the drugs it was prescribing month by month, comparing this with the FHSA average. This was called the 'PACT' data system. It was not enough.

The Treasury had been keen to apply cash limits to drugs spending for a long period; it used the Prime Minister's NHS review to pursue that agenda. The White Paper (Department of Health, 1989a) proposed a system of modified cash limits or 'firm' drugs budgets. In following years the scheme evolved. Government sets targets for each region and each region sets targets for each FHSA. The FHSA then sets an indicative prescribing amount for each of its practices. This is not set in a rigid way but reflects local factors, such as whether a new old persons' home is to open or changes to the particular composition of a local population. The practice would then be expected to keep within that target. If it did not it would receive a visit from the medical adviser to the FHSA and be asked to explain itself. A small percentage of the budget, about 1.5 per cent, is kept back as a reserve to allow for unavoidable overruns. Any practice would have to make a case to their FHSA to increase their limit if a particularly expensive patient or course of treatment could be explained and justified.

There was an indirect financial incentive for non-fundholding practices to keep within their indicative budgets. If the FHSA managed to keep spending below its target, 35 per cent of the sum would be available to finance improvements in primary care in the FHSA.

For fundholders the incentives were to be direct. Included in the fundholders' budget was an element for drugs, set in a similar way to the indicative prescribing amount for other practices. If the practice overspent it could top up with savings from the rest of its budget. If it underspent it could use the savings on another part of the fund. This certainly appealed to most of the GPs we interviewed in the early stages, though some were apprehensive about how the budget would be set.

In what follows we examine what steps our practices took to review their prescribing habits and whether in the end it made any difference to fundholders' drugs spending compared to non-fundholders. First, we consider setting the budgets.

## SETTING GPS' DRUGS BUDGETS

The starting point for the calculations of an FHSA budget is usually the previous year's budget adjusted to take account of price and population changes. The population is weighted to take account of the higher prescribing costs of old people. Sixty-five-year-olds and above are taken to be three times as costly as the under-sixty-fives. This weighting was used between 1991 and 1993. In 1993–4 a more complex weighting system was introduced (see Table 7.1).

From this point on different FHSAs use different approaches. The practices' own past prescribing levels and special factors known to the FHSA are important elements in what is a negotiated settlement. The factors that FHSAs normally take into account are:

● Past levels of practice prescribing.
● An uplift factor for prices and changes in drugs on the market that practices in the area have been using.
● Forecast changes in list size and age–sex balance.

**Table 7.1** The prescribing budget formula

| Age | Patients on list given the following weighting: | |
|---|---|---|
| | Men | Women |
| 0–4 | 1 | 1 |
| 5–14 | 1 | 1 |
| 15–24 | 1 | 2 |
| 25–34 | 1 | 2 |
| 35–44 | 2 | 3 |
| 45–54 | 3 | 4 |
| 55–64 | 6 | 6 |
| 65–74 | 10 | 10 |
| 75 plus | 10 | 12 |
| Temporary residents | 0.5 | 0.5 |

- Changes in the numbers of patients requiring particularly expensive medicines.
- Changes in service provision, for example a new clinic for hypertension.
- Special factors, such as an old persons' home being opened in the practice's area.
- Hospital outpatient prescribing practice.
- Neighbourhood factors.

There is clearly room here for negotiation and judgement.

As the calculation of next year's budget began from the previous year's total, one intending fundholder in 1990 told us, 'We didn't exactly skimp our prescribing.'

One of our practices had taken part in a special project to examine its prescribing several years previously and was well below the FHSA average when we first saw them. In the year before fundholding their spending rose towards the FHSA average. FHSAs tried to counter such drift but were not entirely successful. Thus the first effect of fundholding may have been to increase drugs expenditure. Nevertheless, subsequent periods have seen the incentives begin to work.

## THE PRACTICES' RESPONSE

The impact of the PACT data on most practices was to make them look more carefully at their prescribing where they appeared to be far above the local average, but the coming of formal indicative budgets for non-fundholders did not seem to have changed their approach noticeably. The inducement to prescribe less for the vague benefit of primary care in the area generally simply had no impact. 'There would be no guarantee we would benefit as a result of holding back, why should our patients suffer for no likely gain?' This was a typical response.

From the fundholders the response was different. Most of our group of first-wave practices initially felt they might make some savings on their drugs budget and use the savings to supplement the rest of their budget. The most obvious way of doing this seemed to be to review the partners' use of generic drugs and see if it could be boosted. Another fairly straightforward starting point was to ask the GPs to keep a close watch on repeat prescriptions. A third was to do a careful trawl through their PACT data to see if they could detect exceptional trends with the help of the FHSA medical adviser. None of this was new but it was given an added impetus by the hope that the practices might make savings for their own benefit. A minority of the practices took really major steps to revise their drugs policy as a direct result of becoming fundholders.

One had a list size of 13,500 and several branch surgeries. The partners decided to institute a practice formulary. Once a fortnight one of the partners would present a 'drugs audit', analysing with the help of the computerized records the practice's prescribing habits. Options for the most cost-effective alternatives were presented and discussed bearing in mind patient acceptability and hospital consultant practice. After each meeting a policy was drawn up for the practice on that range of drugs. Each partner was given a copy of the recommendations and had it on their personal computer. Each partner continued to have clinical freedom to prescribe as they wished but the fact that all participated in drawing up the recommendations meant that they were largely followed. It had reduced the range of drugs used and reminded GPs of the generic alternatives. No patient received supplies for more than 30 days and repeat prescriptions were monitored very closely. A course of treatment requiring repeats was entered on the computer, the patient given a slip with dates marked and ticked off each time. A review by the GP was required at a given point.

In the first full year of operating this system the practice managed to reduce its drugs spend below the cash limit by £44,000. Another two practices had followed the policy almost exactly, though with less success in terms of savings.

Other practices listed the most common drugs prescribed and the costs of alternatives. Others had done a less exhaustive audit of the most expensive drugs and their alternatives and reviews of the most commonly prescribed drugs and their alternatives.

It seems clear, therefore, that the direct financial incentives fundholders had to save on their drugs budgets did change their prescribing procedures. The impact on spending was less clear and more complicated.

Hospitals, too, were under pressure and they responded by cost shifting. Hospital consultants determine the drugs regime under which discharged patients live. This can be for a few weeks or many years. To save their hospitals' budgets, consultants limited the drugs they gave patients to take home to a week's supply. The GPs then had to pick up the consequences, continuing to prescribe the drugs. This was of course true for fundholders and non-fundholders alike, but the former were directly losing money as a result. The shorter stays by patients in hospital had the same effect. Hospital consultants are therefore in a free good situation. It does not greatly matter to them if they prescribe an expensive drug, their budget will not suffer, much, and the fundholding GPs will have to pay.

Our GPs argued that consultants hardly ever prescribed a generic drug. They often prescribed a very expensive new alternative to a very similar if slightly less effective drug. In some cases the GPs took this up with the consultant concerned but had little leverage over him or her. The growing prescription of fertility drugs by consultants was causing concern. They are expensive and the courses of treatment long. One group of fundholders pooled all their expertise and negotiated a hospital contract for fertility treatment that specified the drugs regime and the length of treatment.

The NHS centrally began to recognize that there was a problem for all GPs in consultant prescribing and issued a letter of advice to districts (EL(91)127) suggesting that they make this issue part of their contract negotiations. It is, however, of no direct importance to districts in the way it is to GPs and especially fundholding GPs and little seems to have happened.

For a GP the impact of a single, high-cost patient can be significant. One practice had three cardiac transplant patients, a liver transplant patient, a renal transplant and one on growth hormone replacement therapy. The average monthly cost per transplant patient was £750. The total quarterly cost for the six patients was £14,000. They took about 2 per cent of the total drugs budget but were 0.00034 per cent of the practice population!

Basic social factors were pushing up demand as well as changing hospital practice. Patients were much more aware of the existence of hormone replacement therapy, anti-hypertension agents, fertility drugs, steroid inhalers for asthma and many more. The practices were running more screening clinics for hypertension in response to the inducements in the new contract for health promotion and Health of the Nation targets. These tended to push up the drugs bill.

All in all, despite considerable efforts to contain their drugs spending most of our practices ended by overspending their drug budgets, some quite substantially. The overspends were often met out of underspends on the hospital budgets (see Chapter 8). Nevertheless, local information suggested that our practices had been more successful than non-fundholders in limiting the growth of their prescribing. National data and other studies confirmed this impression.

## THE OUTCOME

We were not in a position to be able to undertake a detailed examination of the prescribing changes as they affected patients. Nor did we have a control group of practices from which we could collect prescribing costs. However, other studies of this kind have been undertaken and the results published.

Burr *et al*. (1992) undertook a survey of four fundholders' and four non-fundholders' prescribing in Mid-Glamorgan. They concluded, that although 'fundholders do not appear averse to the introduction of new and more expensive treatments they still managed to reduce their expenditure on drugs in a rational manner', and 'such changes in prescribing patterns as adopted by the fundholders were unlikely to be detrimental to patient care'.

Two larger control trials were reported in late 1993 (Bradlow and Coulter, 1993; Maxwell *et al*., 1993). Angela Coulter's research group in Oxfordshire compared prescribing costs in fundholding and non-fundholding practices before and after the reforms took effect. They studied three dispensing fundholding practices and five non-dispensing ones alongside seven non-dispensing non-fundholding practices. Data was obtained for two six-month periods in 1990–1 and 1991–2.

Prescribing costs increased in all the practices between the two periods but the increase was less for the fundholders. The net cost for dispensing fundholders rose 10.2 per cent and for non-dispensing fundholders by 13.2 per cent. The comparable rise for non-fundholders was 18.7 per cent. The average cost per item showed a more marked differential, suggesting that the fundholders were achieving their lower costs by going for cheaper drugs to a significant extent, bearing out our observations. The increase in the average cost per item for dispensing fundholders was 4.8 per cent and 5.3 per cent for the rest; non-fundholders' increase in cost per item was 11.9 per cent. Contrary to our findings however, five of the fundholders made savings on their drugs budgets rather than over-spending.

Using a different methodology Professor Howie's team in Edinburgh came to similar conclusions (Maxwell *et al.*, 1993). Their practices were taking part in a shadow fundholding project. Their prescribing was analysed using the defined daily dose measure. They concluded that during the two years studied both sets of practices had reduced their volume of prescribing for the classes of drugs they were analysing. Unit costs rose but the fundholding practices managed to hold down this increase more successfully. Unit costs rose in the fundholding practices by 24 per cent and by 11 per cent and 16 per cent in the fundholding areas.

These small-scale studies are in line with the national figures. In 1991–2 all GPs in the country prescribed 15 per cent more in cost terms than the year before; the fundholders' increase was 12 per cent. In 1992–3 the gap was wider; the national average increase in prescribing costs was 12 per cent but the fundholders' increase was only 8 per cent in 1992–3. The projected overspend by non-fundholding GPs on their indicative budgets was 9 per cent; for fundholders the figure was 1.4 per cent. One survey in the North Western Region by the Medicines Resources Centre showed that fundholders make much more use of generic drugs (*Fundholding*, 21 May 1993).

In short, the imposition of a cash limit on fundholders' drugs budgets does seem to have had the intended effect of containing their prescribing more than the arrangements for non-fundholders. If there are to be cash limits on NHS expenditure, and this is inevitable, the case for applying them to all spending is powerful. Not to do so results in resources flowing to the non-cash-limited services for no other reason than administrative chance. A means of applying cash limits that enables professionals to make priority decisions between types of spending and to think hard about their spending priorities must be desirable. The fundholders in our study do seem to have responded in this way.

# 8

# MANAGING THE BUDGET

Contracting with hospitals was a net addition to GPs' powers and the practices mostly relished it, despite the extra work it brought. Handling their own budget was the aspect of the scheme that GPs were most apprehensive about in our initial interviews in 1990. Practices would have to keep within a cash limit. They would have to do the priority setting, the saying no. This was all new territory and would mean an unknown amount of work. Nevertheless, this was the practices' money, or so they saw it; it was jealously husbanded. In the four years of our study we experienced the heady atmosphere of the meetings at the practice (and, often, the local fundholding group), discussing strategy and tactics, the hard bargaining on budgets with representatives from the RHA and the FHSA, the long negotiations with managers and consultants from the local hospital. We describe the way budgets were set and what we think is wrong with the method in Chapter 9. In this chapter we are concerned with the way the practices themselves managed their budgets.

Most of the key partners and practice managers who took part in the budget setting and contracting negotiations found them fascinating and rewarding, if frustrating at times. It left them with a sense of excitement and empowerment. In contrast the process of running the budgets was something of an anti-climax. Most of the GPs themselves wanted to have very little to do with this aspect and sought to employ a new, or train an existing, practice manager. Some practice managers grew marvellously into their new roles over the four years we watched them. Some could not, and left to be replaced by someone with accounting or management experience who had been running a small business or who had been working in a local hospital.

**Table 8.1**  Financial reports submitted to the FHSA

| Report | Content | Frequency |
| --- | --- | --- |
| Statement 1 | Income and expenditure account | Monthly |
| Statement 2 | Savings account | Monthly |
| Statement 3 | Balance sheet | Monthly |
| Statement 4 | Income and expenditure and FHSA payments forecast | Monthly |
| Statement 5 | Cash payments analysis | Annually |
| Schedule 1 | Hospital services expenditure summary | Monthly |
| Schedule 2 | Analysis of proportion of staff costs | Monthly |
| Schedule 3 | Analysis of public sector debtors and creditors | Monthly |
| Schedule 4 | Analysis of private sector debtors and creditors | Monthly |
| Schedule 5 | Analysis of other current assets | Monthly |
| Schedule 6 | FHSA account | Monthly |
| Schedule 7 | General Practice current account | Monthly |
| Schedule 8 | Analysis of other current liabilities | Monthly |

## THE FLOW OF FUNDS

Although the overall responsibility for the scheme rests with the Regional Health Authorities, local control is left to the FHSAs. One of the most important tasks of the FHSAs has been to manage the flow of funds. Their function is two-fold:

1 FHSAs are the caretakers of the practices' accounts, paying bills on behalf of the practices, and ensuring that practices are provided with the necessary funds to meet their day-to-day commitments.
2 FHSAs are the controllers of the practices' financial transactions, monitoring expenditure to ensure that funds are spent in accordance with the scheme, and analysing the expenditure and activity returns that practices submit monthly in order to detect possible difficulties.

In view of this, practices are required to submit certain financial reports to their FHSAs. These are listed in Table 8.1.

Monthly reports must be submitted to the FHSA no later than a month from the end of the month to which they refer. In addition to

this, every March, at the end of each financial year, practices have
to 'balance the books' – reporting to their FHSA their total
transactions and final position for the year. In order to do this, they
are asked to submit all the financial reports for the end of the year.
For this, practices are allowed an extra two weeks; the deadline for
submission of annual reports to the FHSAs is 15 May.

Practice budgets originally covered three broad spending areas:
(1) a defined range of hospital services; (2) the cost of all drugs and
appliances; and (3) a proportion of staff costs. Fund management
proved relatively straightforward as regards the drugs and the staff
elements of the budget but is most problematic in respect to hospital
spending.

## The drugs bill

Data on each practice's prescription costs are collected nationally
by the Prescription Pricing Authority (PPA). The authority supplies every practice and its FHSA with a monthly statement,
approximately six weeks in arrears, setting out the practice's
prescribing in that month. The statement shows the total value of
drugs and appliances prescribed and dispensed for the practice and
paid for by the NHS during the relevant month.

The accuracy of the 'prescription analysis and cost' (PACT) data
is generally regarded as excellent. There are several levels of
analysis, breaking down figures by individual doctor, therapeutic
category, drug classification, etc. Comparisons with the practice's
prescription volume and costs in the previous year, as well as with
the national and FHSA average are also provided (we discussed
their use by practices in Chapter 7). PACT data are used by the
FHSA to debit the GP fundholders' fund. Beyond that, all a
practice has to do is to observe accounting conventions, entering the
equivalent amount in its expenditure accounts.

Therefore, managing the flow of funds in relation to prescription
costs is rather uncomplicated, and the administrative effort required by the practice minimal.

## Staff costs

Payments to staff are initially made from the practice's own bank
account. The practice has to collect supporting documentation
(copies of payments, receipts, etc.), and to keep records on the

separate categories of staff costs (salaries, employer's National Insurance contributions, superannuation, holiday pay, sick pay, maternity pay, etc.). Payments are subsequently recharged to the fund account, following which the FHSA reimburses the practice transferring the appropriate amount (equal to 70 per cent of gross salary and 100 per cent of employer's National Insurance contributions) to the practice's own bank account.

Usually, the flow of funds as regards staff payments is smooth and uneventful. The only slight complication arises when staff costs are unknown by the time a month's accounts are closed, in which case the practice is required to make an accrual for the likely costs. The difference between anticipated and actual costs is corrected when the payment is eventually made.

## Hospital costs

If the management of cash flows is relatively straightforward in respect of prescription and staff costs, the management of payments to hospitals for services provided to the practice's patients and covered by the fundholding scheme has been fraught with difficulties.

The transfer of funds to hospitals for services provided to patients of fundholding practices is arranged by the FHSAs. Each time a payment is due, the practice has to authorize its FHSA to forward the relevant amount to the service provider. Practices do not hold funds in their own bank accounts, except for the everyday needs of running the practice.

Despite the fact that hospitals are paid through the FHSAs, the responsibility for managing budget expenditure rests with the practices. As FHSAs can only act on the practices' specific instructions, it is essential that practices themselves keep detailed records of referrals to hospitals. In order to ensure that they only pay for services they have ordered and for which they are liable under the provisions of the scheme, fundholding practices have to check every single invoice sent from service providers.

The contracts that practices can place with hospitals fall broadly into three categories:

1 *Block*. This confers on the purchaser the right of access to the services provided by a hospital, or a particular speciality within the hospital, in return for a previously agreed annual fee.

2 *Cost and volume.* This guarantees that the hospital undertakes to treat a minimum number of the practice's patients in a particular speciality, or will perform a minimum number of a particular procedure in return for a minimum sum. If the specified activity target is exceeded, additional treatments are carried out on a cost per case basis, as below.

3 *Cost per case.* Unlike the previous two kinds of contract, not placed in advance, but as the occasion arises. Refers to specific cases of patients treated at the hospital for a price agreed at the time of the referral.

### Block contracts

From the point of view of administrative convenience, block contracts are the easiest to manage. Under a block contract purchasers only buy access to a facility, payment is not related to actual utilization. Providers invoice the purchaser for the agreed sum, and payments are usually made in monthly instalments. As contract targets do not exist as such, hospital performance against such targets need not be monitored for financial purposes. Deviations from anticipated activity levels can only be taken into account by the contracting parties when negotiations resume, in the following year's round.

### Cost and volume contracts

On the scale of budgetary convenience block contracts are closely followed by cost and volume contracts. These allow providers to send monthly invoices to the practices for one-twelfth of the agreed sum. However, unlike block contracts, cost and volume contracts require that hospital performance is monitored against targets, in order that deviations are cleared at the end of the year.

If targets are exceeded, an additional payment is made for the extra treatments on a cost per case basis. If, on the other hand, activity is below the levels specified in the contracts, as is usually the case, the practice can negotiate a refund, or, at the very least, seek to remedy the situation in the following year. Either way, the close monitoring of hospital performance against targets is necessary. As a result, although payments can go ahead regardless of whether billing is accurate or not, the validity of reports notifying the practice that treatment has been completed and counted towards contract targets needs to be carefully checked by the practice.

## Cost per case

Like cost and volume contracts, activity reports in relation to targets agreed under cost per case contracts need to be scrutinized by the practice. However, in contrast to cost and volume contracts, payment for services covered by the scheme and provided to the patients of a fundholding practice cannot be made unless the practice has been correctly invoiced.

Cost per case contracts allow a degree of flexibility which comes nearest to the concept of a 'spot market' for hospital services, in which practices 'shop around' for 'bargains'. Initially, most practices used cost per case contracts when they referred to hospitals other than their main provider under special circumstances, e.g. to require an uncommon treatment at a specialist centre, to send a patient to a teaching hospital, etc. Nevertheless, an increasing number of practices were using cost per case contracts on a more systematic basis, as we saw in Chapter 6.

Once a referral is made, hospitals are expected to notify practices of the date of booked admission or attendance at an outpatient clinic as soon as this is known. Detailed guidance on how to handle referral information is contained in the manual of guidance from the DoH. Furthermore, hospitals are also required to notify practices when treatment is commenced. Practices must then enter an amount representing anticipated expenditure once such a notification is received. Practices should therefore be able to make an 'accrual' for the expected cost, even before the invoice has been received and a payment has been made. Once a treatment is completed, hospitals are expected to invoice the practice within a month.

The 'accruals' principle, to which fundholding practices are required to adhere, is one of the four fundamental accounting concepts.[1] It specifies that expenditure should be recognized as incurred, and not as money is paid. Beyond accounting convention,

---

[1] The fundamental accounting concepts are set out in the *Statements of Standard Accounting Practice* and are followed in commercial arrangements. The other three fundamental concepts are: the 'going concern', the 'consistency' concept, and the 'prudence' concept.

the 'accruals' principle allows practices to recognize expenditure as soon as a liability to pay has arisen, and to plan accordingly. There are cases, however, when practices only become aware that fundholding hospital services have been provided to a registered patient when an invoice is received. In such cases, practices run the risk of unanticipated expenditure.

The issue of expenditure 'incurred but not reported' was early recognized as one of the potentially greatest accounting and financial problems fundholding practices might face. Weiner and Ferriss (1990) have pointed out that the experience of Health Maintenance Organizations (HMOs) in the United States showed that services provided to HMO members are often not billed for quite some time. As a result, many HMOs believed they were profitable when in fact they were running large deficits not discovered for months. Management decisions based on a misleading and untimely flow of information caused many HMOs to fail.

## EXPENDITURE CONTROL

The issue of unanticipated expenditure underlines the importance of efficient administrative systems in hospitals and practices, and the need to establish good channels of communication between them. In reality, practices proved much more adaptable than hospitals to the novel requirements of activity recording and contract monitoring which the NHS reforms introduced.

### Hospital expenditure

Hospital administration systems were slow off the mark. In the period immediately after the introduction of the NHS internal market, hospitals were able to carry on very much as before, courtesy of thoughtful district health authorities, who placed block contracts covering the bulk of hospital activities. There was really no difference between the hospital's old budget and a new block contract as far as financial systems were concerned. As a result, most hospitals were not able to deliver the financial and activity data by practice needed to invoice fundholding practices, at least not before hospital managers realized the potential loss of earned revenue involved.

It was no surprise, therefore, that many hospital managers

resented the fact that transactions with fundholding practices, who accounted for only a small proportion of hospitals' revenues, made necessary a complete overhaul of the hospitals' mode of operation, as far as activity records were concerned. The fact that such change was long overdue did not always convince those who insisted that fundholding took up a 'disproportionate amount of hospital resources'.

The disruptive potential to fundholding practices of these administrative difficulties should not be underestimated. Practices reported serious problems with the quality of activity reports sent by hospitals. Errors were common and persistent. One of the practices taking part in our study reported that well into the second year of the scheme 'the error proportion in invoices reached 50 per cent'. The quality of invoicing was 'appalling' said another doctor. Every month his staff had to spend 'a whole week or more' checking the accuracy of bills. The manager of yet another practice told us that it had been 'a few months' before she was able to pass on for payment one single invoice without sending it back to the hospital.

It was often the case that everything that could go wrong with hospital bills *did* go wrong. Practices were billed for procedures that were not covered by the scheme, or for patients who did not belong to them. Often, hospitals inadvertently 'double-charged' practices, for example for outpatient consultations which, according to the contract, should be included in the inpatient price. On other occasions, claims against practice budgets were made for treatments attracting special funding under the national waiting list initiative.

On the other hand, it would be unfair to suggest that errors were all one way: often, invoices missed out treatments already carried out by the hospital and for which practices were liable, just because consultants failed to inform administrators, or because activity went unnoticed by the finance department.

As a result of the inability of hospitals to cope with the requirements of fundholding contracts, practices found they had to spend a greater than expected amount of time on running the scheme in the first year, especially. Invoicing had improved markedly by the third wave but most of the practices in our study had been unable to persuade hospitals to do much about the quality of reports.

Practices found this extremely frustrating and a terrible waste of time. They also found it quite mystifying. 'It is in their interest to get it right after all', they would often say. Practices, not without some pride, compared the speed with which they had adapted to the demands of the new system with what they saw as persistent underperformance on the part of hospitals. They were quite amused to discover that many hospitals relied on the practices to tell them how much they owed them.

Our practices paid hospital bills they knew were outstanding even if the hospital had not claimed them, not least because it would otherwise lead to an unreal underspend, which Region might use to cut their budget next year. One practice told us how, at the end of the year, they had found out that some of their patients had been treated at a well-known teaching hospital which had never sent them an invoice. The practice did not hesitate to send a cheque, together with a mildly ironic letter calling for closer co-operation in the coming year. 'Hospitals are like oil tankers,' reflected a doctor, 'they take three miles to turn around.'

## Software systems

The poor quality of the invoices sent from hospitals was not the only source of frustration for practice staff responsible for day-to-day administration. The fundholding software system used to run the accounts was another.

The specification of the system had been designed in detail by the DoH in the run-up to the reforms. The intention of the DoH was to ensure that the information systems used by fundholding practices followed a standard format, including a minimum set of features necessary for auditing the scheme. In the introduction to the *General Practice Fundholders' Manual of Accounts* (Department of Health, 1990), it was explained that in order 'to assist practices participating in the scheme, the Department produced a computer software specification to enable suppliers of GP computer systems to develop software to assist practices in the production of the necessary financial and management information'. Indeed, several companies brought to the market their competing versions, all carrying DoH approval, and it was agreed that practices would receive 100 per cent reimbursement for the costs involved in purchasing software (about £10,000 to £12,500).

The software packages were all designed to function as accounting systems. This, as described before, was the expressed intention of the DoH. Against this criterion, all of the software packages eventually approved performed adequately. Nevertheless, as the systems were not intended for use as management information systems, they failed to provide practices with speedy answers to the simplest of enquiries on financial transactions, patient flows, etc. As a result, a wealth of important information, which could be used in the day-to-day running of the scheme by practices, remained just beyond the reach of practices. It was not long before the limitations of the fundholding software systems became obvious.

Lack of integration between the fundholding and clinical software systems was the most serious of these limitations. As a result, data on transactions had to be entered twice. Some of the software systems had already been integrated by 1993 and others would be. This problem was an inevitable consequence of the speed of introducing the whole reform, not a long-term problem. Again initially, hospital computing systems were unable to recognize the unique identification number that the fundholding software generated every time a referral was made. Moreover, the system proved to be extremely inflexible. When data on a new transaction were entered, all corresponding entries were also made automatically. However, if a change was necessary, for example because a patient received a different procedure from that envisaged originally, the system would prevent amendments. The original entries had all to be cancelled manually, and new entries had to be made from the start.

Practices were also irritated by the amount of what they saw as unnecessary extra work involved in recording repeat outpatient appointments or pathology requests. Practices gradually learned how 'to trick the system', for example by entering all the pathology requests of the month under the identification number of one imaginary 'patient'. The authorities were notified of and accepted such manoeuvres.

The fundholding software seemed unable to combine in some intelligent manner the information stored in it. For example, confronted with the simple question 'How many of my patients have had a hip replacement in hospital $X$ over the last six months?' all it could manage was a multi-page print-out of all the operations in all hospitals, which doctors had then to analyse manually. Similarly, the system was unable to tell practices how many patients were still waiting for treatment, having been referred to hospital. Nor, for that matter, could it work out what the practice's waiting list was, by hospital and by treatment.

The practices that participated in our study found it invariably disappointing and frustrating that the system could not be used as a management tool. It had been a 'missed opportunity' said a doctor. The fundholding software was 'accountant-friendly but doctor-hostile' quipped another. Most of the practices had to design simple spreadsheets themselves in order to keep track of the information necessary for managing the fund. They all thought the DoH should have known better.

In fact, feedback from fundholding practices did reach the DoH, which, in December 1991, held a meeting with representatives from the RHAs to discuss possible improvements to the software specifications. The meeting concluded that changes aimed to improve communication between hospitals and practices depended on the integration of their information systems, and would take several years to bring about.

However, simpler changes were identified, and the DoH undertook to direct the computer companies to amend their models accordingly. The upgraded versions only became available well into the second year, and suppliers took the opportunity to include provisions for the incorporation from 1993–4 of community health services into the scope of the scheme.

The use of two different software versions in one financial year caused an astonishing degree of disruption. Some practices found they were unable to close their accounts at the end of the second year, in May 1993. First-wave practices were better prepared after a similar experience with an equally chaotic end of year in 1992, but the fact that the software continued to cause problems despite the experience of the initial phase was viewed by all with dismay.

**Administrative costs**

In the light of the above, practices soon realized it was impossible to accommodate the administrative burden of the scheme without organizational changes. Most had to appoint extra clerical staff to do exclusively fundholding work. Furthermore, fund administration required a considerable amount of the practice manager's time. Moreover, partners often found they had to get themselves personally involved in fund management on a regular basis.

Table 8.2 shows the time requirements of fundholding in the ten practices participating in our study. Figures were derived from the

**Table 8.2** Time requirements of fundholding in ten practices

| Practice | Doctor (hours per week) | Management (full-time equivalent) | Clerical (full-time equivalent) |
|----------|------|------|------|
| 1 | 4 | 0.5 | 0.2 |
| 2 | 2 | 0.8 | 1.0 |
| 3 | <1 | 0.5 | 0.5 |
| 4 | 10 | 0.5 | 0.5 |
| 5 | <1 | 0.7 | 1.0 |
| 6 | <1 | 0.8 | 1.5 |
| 7 | 2 | 0.5 | 1.8 |
| 8 | <1 | 0.5 | 1.0 |
| 9 | <1 | 0.5 | 1.0 |
| 10 | 2 | 0.7 | 1.0 |
| Average | 2.25 (approx.) | 0.6 | 0.95 |

replies of partners and practice managers to the relevant questions raised during our interviews.

Table 8.2 demonstrates that day-to-day administration requires between 50 and 80 per cent of a practice manager's time, at an average of 60 per cent. In most cases, managers worked longer following the introduction of fundholding, some up to 55 hours per week. In all practices managers had tried to delegate some of the less demanding aspects of their responsibilities to clerical staff and VDU operators. On average, the full-time equivalent of 0.9 staff was required for data input and computer work, ranging from 0.2 at the smallest of our ten practices to 1.8 at the largest.

For comparison, *Fundholding* magazine is advising practices about to join the scheme that although the time taken up by fundholding varies, and usually depends on a practice's patient list size, as a guide practices should anticipate the need for one to three staff (1 to 1.5 full-time equivalent) to do clerical work, plus one more staff member (0.5 to 1 full-time equivalent) to perform fund management tasks.

The involvement of doctors in day-to-day fund management varied enormously between practices. In five of the ten practices in our study partners had little more to do than 'a bit of extra paperwork' as one doctor put it. In the remaining five practices doctors had to dedicate between two hours per week and two hours per day on administration. It must be stressed that these estimates do not include the amount of managerial time spent by doctors on budget setting and contract negotiations (the highlights in the fundholding calendar), at the beginning of each financial year. The management allowance recognizes this and does allow a locum to be paid for up to half a day a week to replace the time taken by a partner if that is the way a practice wishes to arrange matters at any point.

Practices usually took steps *not* to allow fund administration to get in the way of patient care. Usually, the partner responsible for fundholding simply worked longer in order to catch up with the paperwork. The extra work involved in fundholding began, in some practices, to take a toll.

Half-way through the second year, a partner in one of our smaller practices told us he faced a dilemma between 'letting his list size slip' and 'drastically reducing the amount of time spent on fundholding'. The practice considered the option of employing a full-time manager in place of their existing occasional use of a freelance business consultant, but rejected it on the grounds that 'fundholding work came in waves' and did not justify a full-time position. However, in our subsequent visit to that practice the same doctor told us rather glumly that he had to give up half a day's surgery time per week. In other words, one of his ten weekly sessions had become unavailable for patient consultations. The doctor was worried about the effect of that on his patient list size.

Clearly, this was not an isolated case. Although all practices in our study were determined to get on with the scheme, resentment of the amount of administration involved, and the implications for the time available for ordinary general practice work, was evident. In a visit to another practice, the doctors reported that as a result of fundholding they had to reduce the number of health promotion clinics offered to patients.

Similar findings have been reported elsewhere. In a survey of 128 first-wave fundholding practices (out of a total 306) published in October 1991 in *Fundholding* magazine, 95 per cent of respondents said that participation in the scheme had 'increased their workload'. Almost one-quarter (22 per cent) of practices claimed that fund-holding required an extra 20 hours per week.

Another study of ten first-wave fundholding practices in the Northern Region between March and July 1992 (Newton *et al.*,

1993) asked doctors, managers and other staff to assess their experience of the scheme, and, in particular, the impact of fundholding on patient care and practice management. While doctors and non-clinical staff thought that the benefits outweighed the costs, all respondents perceived 'increased time and effort in administration', or simply 'extra work' as the main disadvantage of fundholding for their practice.

Similarly, a review of five fundholding practices in three English regions (McAvoy, 1993), while discovering a sense of 'real enthusiasm and empowerment' and 'tangible improvements in patient care', also revealed that preparing for and implementing fundholding had been an 'enormous administrative task' in the experience of all doctors interviewed.

The widespread concern of participants in the scheme with the administrative burden it places on practices has not gone unnoticed by opponents of fundholding. In a passionate (and rather apocalyptic) call to non-fundholding practices to remain so indefinitely, an Oxford general practitioner writing in the BMJ listed 'greatly increased administrative workload' as the first of his six 'reasons for not fundholding' (Keeley, 1993).

On the other hand, the best-run of our first-wave practices had settled down to a routine that put fundholding well down the list of their administrative worries by the second year. One manager told us, 'I don't think most of the partners really know it's happening most of the time.' This much more relaxed attitude was more widely shared amongst third-wave practices by the time of our last interviews in mid-1993, their third year. None raised administration as a major worry.

## FINANCIAL RESULTS

How then did the budgets actually work out at the end of the year?

In the first three years of the scheme, as we discuss in detail in Chapter 9, budgets were set on the basis of the previous year's activity levels. Practices were therefore convinced that if they did not spend up to their limit the region would cut their budgets next year. Indeed, many health authorities interpreted the largely unintended underspends caused by hospital inactivity or changed prices as a proof that budgets had been over-generous in the first place. Some practices were ordered to return unspent funds to the local DHA. Most had joined the scheme partly in order to clear the waiting lists and, as a result, thought there was no point in savings. 'Our practice is proud to have treated more patients than ever before' said the manager of such a practice. 'I told the doctors: "spend, spend, spend".'

**Temporal variations**

Whatever the spending strategy of a practice, the difficulties with hospital invoicing was a constraining factor. As described earlier, delays and errors made it difficult for a practice to monitor and manage the flow of funds into hospitals. In most cases, hospitals failed to wake up to the revenue implications of faulty invoicing until the predictable rush late into the financial year.

Moreover, some practices experienced difficulties with hospitals under-performing in terms of meeting activity targets, as stipulated in the contracts. It often took pressure, threats of 'exit', and, in certain cases, the actual removal of patients from the local hospital's waiting lists to be treated elsewhere, before practices managed to begin to hit their target spending in year one.

Finally, as fundholding was a novel experience for general practitioners, some practices were cautious to start with, and only became more relaxed and confident as their familiarity with the scheme grew. As soon as practices felt in control, their referral rates returned to normal levels. The nature of inpatient procedures covered by the scheme (mainly elective surgery) enabled practices to turn up and down the volume of their referrals. In this respect fundholders were in quite a different situation to the HMOs discussed by Weiner and Ferriss (1990). A fundholder lengthens his or her queue or speeds it up as required. As a result of the factors described above, fundholding practices' spending was more heavily weighted towards the end of the financial year. This temporal pattern can be exclusively attributed to hospital spending, as expenditure on drugs and staff was evenly distributed throughout the year.

Table 8.3 shows the (unweighted) mean percentage of funds spent in each quarter on hospital services, drugs, and staff, in the ten practices of our study as a whole. Figures are expressed as a proportion of the 'target', i.e. the relevant fraction of the budget for each point in time. A linear pattern of spending is assumed. In other words, the 'target' is taken to be 25 per cent of the budget in the first quarter, 50 per cent at the end of the second quarter, 75 per cent at

**Table 8.3**  Quarterly budget spending projections for the ten fundholding practices as a whole

| Budget element | End of first quarter (%) | End of second quarter (%) | End of third quarter (%) | End of year (%) |
|---|---|---|---|---|
| Hospital | 52.8 | 73.6 | 85.2 | 91.7 |
| Drugs | 94.6 | 97.7 | 98.8 | 103.1 |
| Staff | 99.3 | 100.3 | 100.6 | 101.2 |
| Total | 72.2 | 84.1 | 91.2 | 96.3 |

the end of the third quarter, and 100 per cent at the end of the year. For convenience, all 'targets' are given in percentage terms.

Table 8.3 shows that, at the end of the first quarter (30 June), practices had spent about half the funds designated for the purchase of hospital services in three months. Had this pattern persisted until the end of the year, practices would have made an underspend of almost 50 per cent. By September, the end of the first six months, hospital invoicing (and with it, spending against budgets) had made up some of the lost ground. Practices had spent on average three-quarters of the half year's share of the hospital budget, and were set to make an underspend of about 25 per cent.

Hospital spending rallied to 85 per cent of budgeted expenditure at the end of the third quarter (31 December), to finish at 92 per cent at the end of the year. Late invoices increased the proportion of actual to budget expenditure on hospital services even further after the end of the year. Considering the difficulties the practices had in getting up-to-date figures from the hospitals and the caution they exhibited in not wanting to overspend, this was a good outcome.

In contrast, expenditure on drugs and staff showed little variation, remaining around the target throughout the year. As a result, average spending as a proportion of the relevant fraction of the total budget at the end of each quarter rose from 72 per cent at the end of June, to 84 per cent at the end of September, to 91 per cent at the end of December and 96 per cent at the end of March.

**Spending by budget element**

Table 8.3 shows that practices underspent their hospital budget and overspent their drugs budget. This is shown more clearly in the

**Table 8.4**   Financial results by budget element for the ten fundholding practices as a whole

| Budget element | Original budget (£) | Final budget (£) | Spending (£) | Variation | |
|---|---|---|---|---|---|
| | | | | £ | % |
| Hospital | 7,855,809 | 7,892,984 | 7,333,325 | 559,659 | 7.1 |
| Drugs | 5,349,853 | 5,309,979 | 5,458,636 | (154,657) | (2.9) |
| Staff | 1,256,000 | 1,273,659 | 1,272,953 | 724 | <0.1 |
| Total | 14,461,662 | 14,470,622 | 14,064,896 | 405,726 | 2.8 |

Brackets = overspending.

financial results by budget element for the ten fundholding practices as a whole, presented in Table 8.4.

Table 8.4 demonstrates that practice accounts showed a 7 per cent underspend in the hospital budget, partly offset by a 3 per cent overspend in the drugs budget. Eight out of ten practices underspent their hospital budget, by up to 21 per cent, while one practice was just above budget (0.3 per cent) and another overspent by 3 per cent. On the other hand, six out of ten practices overspent their drugs budget (by up to 21 per cent in one case, but below 8 per cent in the other five), while four practices underspent, by between 1.3 and 5.5 per cent.

The result of drugs budget overspends and hospital budget underspends was the increased weight of prescription costs in the finances of the ten fundholding practices examined here. While the drugs element of budgets accounted for 36.7 per cent of total *budgets*, drugs *spending* was 38.8 per cent of total spending. On the other hand, hospital services accounted for 54.6 per cent of total budgets, but only for 52.1 per cent of total spending.

This small but significant shift in emphasis had not been anticipated by the practices. Indeed, as we saw, most practices had hoped to reduce the cost of their prescriptions. We discussed some of the reasons for this in Chapter 7.

### Spending by practice

The end of first year results for each of the ten practices of our study are presented in Table 8.5. On joining the scheme, practices were

**Table 8.5**    Financial results for each of the ten fundholding practices

| Practice | Original budget (£) | Final budget (£) | Spending (£) | Difference £ | Difference % |
|---|---|---|---|---|---|
| 1 | 999,971 | 885,551 | 771,680 | 113,871 | 12.9 |
| 2 | 1,807,918 | 1,807,918 | 1,846,255 | (38,337) | (2.1) |
| 3 | 1,791,425 | 1,829,726 | 1,809,395 | 20,331 | 1.1 |
| 4 | 1,526,348 | 1,549,348 | 1,528,337 | 21,011 | 1.4 |
| 5 | 984,000 | 1,035,710 | 960,212 | 75,498 | 7.3 |
| 6 | 1,320,000 | 1,326,079 | 1,386,151 | (60,072) | (4.5) |
| 7 | 1,416,000 | 1,416,000 | 1,421,604 | (5,604) | (0.4) |
| 8 | 1,172,000 | 1,172,000 | 988,627 | 183,373 | 15.6 |
| 9 | 1,800,000 | 1,804,290 | 1,786,388 | 17,902 | 1.0 |
| 10 | 1,644,000 | 1,644,000 | 1,566,247 | 77,753 | 4.7 |
| All | 14,461,662 | 14,470,622 | 14,064,896 | 405,726 | 2.8 |

Brackets = overspending.

given budgets of between £1 million and £1.8 million each. One practice had more than £110,000 returned to the health authorities in the middle of the year, as a result of errors made in the calculation of the hospital budget. Similar errors, but in the opposite direction, and other unforeseen factors led to further allocations of funds totalling about £120,000 to five more practices.

It can be seen that in five of these practices the deviation of actual from budgeted spending was rather small (from between 1.4 per cent below budget to 2.1 per cent above budget). Only one practice registered a substantial overspend of 4.5 per cent. The remaining four practices underspent by between 4.7 and 15.6 per cent. Overall, out of a total £14.5 million allocated to the ten practices, a combined underspend of £400,000 (2.8 per cent of total budgets) was made. In view of the fact that the ten practices covered a population of 125,000 between them, their average underspend in the first year of the scheme was just above £3 per patient.

Data from the three regional health authorities covered by our study suggest that the experience of the ten practices examined here was not unrepresentative of other fundholding practices in their area.

## CONCLUSIONS

Despite the fears many practices had before the scheme began it proved easier to keep within the limits of the budgets than critics had supposed. Practices, dealing only with non-emergency cases, had been able to speed up or slow down the flow of patients to keep within budget. The main difficulty had been hospitals' incapacity to provide up-to-date billing information and changes in price levels after the budget had been set. In the second and third years things had gone more smoothly in this respect. Billing had been a big administrative change for practices but overall an outsider can only wonder that the change was carried through as smoothly as it was. Corroborating evidence for this is the number of practices who were going for case by case billing by the third wave.

In short, all the dire predictions of bankruptcy and financial incompetence that had been so widespread when we began the research were simply unfounded. The practices had shown themselves a good deal more financially adept and attuned to the new market world than districts or hospitals. On reflection this was not so surprising. GPs are after all small business people, and are used to managing their own financial affairs in a market place.

# 9

# BUDGET SETTING

## SETTING THE FIRST BUDGET

How to set the budgets the GPs were to spend? This turned out to be the most difficult and contentious element in the whole story.

The Government had begun with the belief that the fundholding budgets could be set in much the same way as districts' – a payment for each patient enrolled on their list (Department of Health, 1989). The payments would be varied to take account of such factors as old people making more use of hospital services, for example. However, it was soon clear it was just not that simple. In the first place there was no way of knowing what factors to build into such a formula. Clearly old people would make more use of hospital services covered by the fund, but how much more? How much more expensive would women be? What about high-cost, chronically ill patients? We discuss these issues in detail in Chapter 10. Here it is enough to note that the DoH's officials soon abandoned the idea of trying to concoct a formula for the first-wave practice budgets. What were they to do instead?

The primary goal was to ensure that GPs were attracted to the scheme and that they would not have to disrupt their existing patterns of care or usage of hospitals. The aim was still minimum disruption – the steady state. The way to do this, it was finally concluded, was to set the budgets so that they would enable GPs to buy the same number of treatments of the same kind from the same hospitals as they always had. If they wished to spend their budgets differently that would be acceptable, but the cash they were given should be enough to preserve their traditional referral pattern and scale.

Regions would therefore set the budget by finding out how many patients had been referred to which hospital and then multiplying these activity rates by the prices charged in these hospitals speciality by speciality.

That sounded simple enough. There were regional statistics on hospital activity and which GP had referred the patients – a computer search should be enough, we were told in early 1990. Not so. The regional computer-based returns from hospitals only covered *inpatient* services. Outpatients were a large part of the budget and no one knew at Region where the patients came from. The handwritten records were unreliable. So too, it turned out, were the computer records for inpatients. On top of this the information was out of date – by up to two years. The new Korner system of statistical returns health authorities are obliged to make to central government was not yet adapted to meet these needs either. The region had no option but to ask the practices themselves to fill in returns from their own records saying where their patients had been referred and treated.

This method had serious disadvantages. It was in the practices' interests to inflate these returns. They had to be put together from different sources (medical records, discharge letters) and done manually. As this was a huge task and had to be done quickly, there was no way records could be produced for the whole past year from most practices. A period of three months had to do in some cases. Were those three months typical of the whole year? The classifications needed were often at odds with the way the practice records were kept. The returns were going to be far from perfect.

To minimize potential bias, the regions pulled together what independent data they could. Region B created a database with information from intending fundholders. Region C used its existing information system on referrals, as did Region A. Where major disparities emerged between the practices' returns and these other sources, the practice was challenged and its figures cross-checked. The difficulty was that the hospital data were often shown to be poor – perhaps only half the referrals having a GP's name attached. Some of the practices had very good computerized patient information and they could successfully challenge the regional officers.

When the practices' referral and activity rates had been settled there was another problem. What price would the hospitals charge? This was the first year of pricing and hospitals were struggling to come up with any prices. Regions gave guidance but local providers

**Table 9.1**   Fundholding budgets per patient in the three regions, 1991–2

| Region | Hospital (£) | Drugs (£) | Total (£) |
|---|---|---|---|
| A | 56.61 (10.12) | 33.08 (8.77) | 99.02  (7.43) |
| B | 64.67 (11.29) | 38.44 (5.37) | 111.19 (13.31) |
| C | 59.79  (8.52) | 46.93 (7.68) | 116.46 (15.02) |
| All three RHAs | 61.20 (10.73) | 38.61 (8.61) | 108.61 (13.71) |

The figures in parentheses are standard deviations.

did not necessarily follow it. The DoH had recommended that hospitals use average speciality costs as a starting point weighting, this to take account of treatments that might involve long stays.

What prices would the regions use in setting the practices' budgets though? Many providers were nowhere near ready to set their prices by the time the budgets had to be set. For this reason two regions decided to fix the budgets using a regional costing model and hoping the eventual prices would not be very different. The third region asked provider units and trusts to estimate prices for themselves. Business plans had to include a price list.

Outpatient costs were a further problem. Two regions used an average cost per referral. The other region favoured attendance as the unit. It took outpatient expenditure in each speciality and divided by the number of attendances.

Diagnostic tests involved a different calculation. One region used average costs across all kinds of pathology tests. Another distinguished the types of test requested by the practices in the past.

The final difficulty was that the regions could not be sure the prices they had assumed hospitals would charge would actually be charged to particular practices.

Many budgets were over- or under-calculated for this reason and had to be recalculated afterwards when the prices became clear. Practices were quick to complain if the prices set were higher than those used in the calculation but were reluctant to 'give back' money when the mistake had gone the other way.

In the end, the budgets set for the first-wavers were accepted by the practices. Few practices left the scheme on their account. The scheme was off to a reasonable start. The precedents set. The problems would come later.

The budgets worked out at just over £100 per patient, or £1

million for a practice with 10,000 patients (Table 9.1). Though the regional averages were reasonably close, the variations between practices were quite wide. In Region B the lowest budget per patient was £85 and the highest £137. This variability was not, of course, the result of fundholding. It merely put £ signs on the wide variation in referral patterns we already knew existed (Roland *et al.*, 1990).

## SETTING THE BUDGETS FOR THE SECOND TIME

In the second year the task began to escalate. Budgets for the first wave had to be rolled forward and new ones set for the second wave. The question was 'Had last year's budget been set appropriately?' As the scheme was set to grow, the significance of this question also began to grow. The impact on district budgets would grow from the odd percentage point to a major slice they would lose to the practices. Regional officers were under pressure from their colleagues to contain the rise. Moreover, in the run-up to negotiations in the first quarter of 1992 there was a widespread belief among regional officers that first-year budgets *had* been too generous. In the words of one, 'Last year the main worry of the Region was to give fundholders enough, not realizing that there was actually a risk of giving too much.' As most first-wave practices in the three regions had indeed been able to make some savings in the first year of the scheme, regional officers were faced with the urgent problems of how to treat these savings and, in the light of that, how to set second-year budgets.

The DoH had advised regions to differentiate between fortuitous and efficiency savings. Savings resulting from a provider setting lower prices from the ones used to calculate budgets were indefensible. These had mostly been clawed back during the first year. However, if a practice 'shopped around' for lower prices, switching referral patterns from one hospital to another in order to achieve lower spending, the resulting savings should be regarded as a reward for 'efficiency gain'. To ask practices to return these savings to the RHA would be to eliminate all incentives for better performance. Regions should see that the efforts of practices were not wasted. At the same time, they should ensure that unfair financial gains were prevented. It was an unenviable task.

The three RHAs all decided that it would be difficult and

undesirable to ask for end-of-year savings to be returned. The aim would be to try to prevent unjustified savings being incorporated into subsequent years. They developed different strategies to deal with the problem of how to sort out 'fortuitous' from 'efficiency' savings.

Region B tried to distinguish 'windfall' savings from 'managed' ones before it allowed the previous year's spend to become the next year's starting point. Regional officers held a series of review meetings and budget negotiations with each practice individually. The Region's method was to compare the number of inpatients actually treated by each practice with the planned number that was incorporated in the previous year's budgets.

The resulting budget offers focused on 'purchasing power', as money used by providers was down in the second year and the intention was to reduce budgets accordingly. On the other hand, this was election year and the Government had given the NHS as a whole the largest increase in funds for a very long time. Nor could officers afford a damaging row in the run-up to an election.

Region A also started from the premise that first-year budgets had been excessive. Regional fundholding officers were determined to be more tight-fisted in the second year. Instead of trying to sort out efficiency savings according to the instructions of the DoH, they followed a simpler rule to link first-year spending with second-year budgets: if savings were under 2 per cent of last year's budget, this year's allocation remained the same as the year before – before the addition of an inflation 'uplift factor', and the usual allowance for list size increases.

On the other hand, if savings were over 5 per cent of budget, the new budget was set equal to what the practice had spent in year one. For example, if last year's budget was £1 million and the practice had spent £0.9 million, this year's budget would be set at £0.9 million (plus the usual adjustments). Savings between 2 and 5 per cent of budget fell in a 'grey area'. Practices in this range were treated individually. Officers admitted that, basically, if a practice 'made a lot of fuss' they kept their underspend.

Region C faced a series of computing problems that did not allow a clear picture of first-year savings to emerge in time for budget negotiations. In the end, the three regions differed considerably in their capacity to hold down the incremental growth from year one to year two. Region A *reduced* the first-wave hospital budgets by 5.5 per cent. The overall budgets were held constant in cash terms. This at a time when the NHS budget as a whole was *rising* by over 5 per cent, and the prescribing budget by much more than that. Region B's budgets rose by 8 per cent and Region C's by nearly 10 per cent, though the hospital element was increased by less than that.

## Setting budgets for second-wave practices

Second-wave budgets in 1992–3 were set as in the year before, on the basis of past patterns of service use. Once more, regions had: (1) to identify what these patterns were; and (2) to establish provider prices for these services. Budgets would be set at a level that enabled practices to purchase their 'usual' mix of hospital services.

Region C was able to use its regional statistical information to obtain inpatient and day case activity by practice. Data on outpatients were derived from the hospital-based Patient Administration Systems.

On the other hand, the spread of self-governing hospitals began to complicate the process of price disclosure for the purposes of budget-setting in most regional health authorities. Many trusts decided, for what they called 'commercial reasons', to withhold information until it was almost too late for setting fundholding budgets. However, this practice was not observed in Region C, where all price lists arrived at the desk of the regional officer in charge of budget setting by early February. This enabled final offers to be made to practices by mid-February, exactly as planned. The offers were better received by practices. The negotiations were conducted without serious problems. There were only four new second-wave practices in the whole region.

In Region A, the process of setting the budgets was almost identical with the year before, only better organized. Practices were asked to collect referral information in the nine-month period of April to December 1991. The RHA did the analysis of crude data.

Practices were given more information in budget presentations (price spreadsheets, etc.). The assumptions used to derive budgets (e.g. the estimated percentage of non-attendances used to convert referral data to activity data in outpatients) were also explained. The whole process was described as 'very comfortable'. Practices were reassured that if prices changed the RHA would provide the extra funding required and they accepted the budget offers more promptly than the year before.

Budgets for second-wave practices in Region A were at reasonable levels in 1992–3. In total, such practices received £105 for each patient compared with £100 per patient for first-wave practices. Hospital budgets, which are to a certain extent controlled by the Region, were at £48 per patient on average, i.e. £6 below the amount granted to the first wave. It was drugs budgets (that lie beyond the Region's jurisdiction) that reversed the picture: the second wave were offered £47 per patient for drugs alone, compared with only £36 awarded to first-wave practices. These increases reflected increased prescribing costs in both fundholding and non-fundholding practices.

In Region B, the whole process of budget-setting encountered more difficulties. The new practices were asked to collect data for six months (April to September) for referrals to inpatients, day cases, outpatients, and requests to direct access, pathology, X-rays, etc. A standard format was required, but not all practices followed this. Data came in all formats: computer discs, standard forms, plain paper, etc. Some practices managed only three months' data, others sent information in a way that was incompatible with that of hospital data collection systems.

There were problems of interpretation of these data. Fundholders are only responsible for what is called 'primary procedures'. Therefore, if a patient is treated for a condition different from, but related to, the one for which he or she was originally referred, this secondary procedure is performed free of charge to the practice, as the cost falls on the district health authority where the patient is resident. Practices instead recorded all treatments separately, which complicated matters enormously.

Practice data were subsequently sent to providers and district health authorities for validation. Districts were unhappy with what they saw as excessive levels of referrals. Although such an attitude was predictable in view of the implications of fundholding for the districts' own budgets, the RHA thought that their case was a genuine one. However, proving it was difficult.

Hospitals under-recorded activity by 50 per cent. In order to get around this, the regional officers turned to the regional database. This again was imperfect, as many service items provided to patients were impossible to attribute to the referring practices.

Using the best data they could muster, officers concluded that, compared to the regional average, the level of referrals was high. A high-level meeting at the RHA took the decision to 'cap' referral

**Table 9.2**   Fundholding budgets per patient in the three regions, 1992–3

| Region | Hospital (£) | Drugs (£) | Total (£) |
|---|---|---|---|
| A | 51.29  (6.54) | 40.33 (10.32) | 102.16 (11.14) |
| B | 68.82 (12.85) | 44.38  (7.03) | 123.24 (16.35) |
| C | 65.37 (13.16) | 54.41  (7.92) | 131.86 (18.93) |
| All three RHAs | 63.18 (13.63) | 45.05  (9.36) | 118.78 (18.49) |

The figures in parentheses are standard deviations.

rates to 57 out of 1000 inpatient referrals and 160 out of 1000 outpatient referrals. No first-wave practices had exceeded these levels. Differences in case mix were not taken into account.

The RHA announced this decision in a letter signed by the finance director of the RHA. The Region admitted that the ceiling was a 'blunt instrument to tackle a complex problem', but said it was prepared to back up practices with additional resources if they got into difficulties.

The other side of the calculation also proved more difficult as more providers became trusts. Providers did not want fundholders to know their provisional price lists. They feared that that might prejudice any subsequent revisions. The trusts kept their cards close to their chests. As late as February two major provider units had not given RHAs any prices. When information did start to flow in, prices changed every week.

In the end, budgets to second-wave practices in Region B were 5 per cent higher than those given to first-wave practices. The former received about £127 for each patient, the latter only £120. Hospital budgets accounted for most of the difference: the second wave was offered £5 more per patient than first-wave practices.

Table 9.2 shows budget allocations per capita to fundholding practices in all three regions in the second year of the scheme.

Budget variations between individual practices were greater than in the first year. The standard deviations increased in all regions (with the exception of hospital budgets in Region A). While total budgets varied from £76 to £172 per patient (a high/low ratio of 2.3), hospital budgets ranged from below £40 to £104 per patient (a high/low ratio of 2.6).

Concerns about the whole process became acute in the third year.

**THE THIRD YEAR (1993–4)**

In 1993–4 the scheme really took off. In the three regions as a whole, the number of participating practices rose, from 44 in 1991–2 and 79 in 1992–3, to 188 in 1993–4. The proportion of residents registered with fundholding practices in the three regions increased from 5.5 per cent in the first year and 10 per cent in the second, to reach 21.3 per cent in the third year.

The great increase in the number of participating practices clearly amounted to a significant claim on the (already stretched) administrative resources of the regional health authorities. However, the large number of new recruits to the scheme was not the only new factor compared to the year before. In 1993, community services' budgets had to be included and more hospitals were now trusts. The DoH was anxious to encourage regions to move to a formula basis for funding (see Chapter 10). Region B, with most GP fundholders, took formula funding most seriously.

**Budget setting in Region B**

The Region includes a county with one of the highest concentrations of fundholding practices in the country. In 1991–2, the practices joining the scheme accounted between them for 15 per cent of the county's population, that is, three times the national average. The following year this proportion doubled to 30 per cent. In 1993–4, exactly 50 per cent of the Region's population found themselves registered with a fundholding practice.

By the time budget setting for the third year of the scheme came to the Region's agenda, a total of 45 practices were getting ready for fundholding in that year, added to the 43 that carried on from the previous years. Moreover, it appeared that hospital activity rates grew higher and higher the more recently the practice joined the scheme. Hospital referrals leading to admission per 1000 population were 43 for the first wave, 48 for the second wave and, according to the preliminary data then available, as high as 57 for the third wave. The resource implications of these rates were clearly immense.

This prospect rang alarm bells. Districts reported that the anticipated transfer of funds from their budgets to those of fundholders would leave them with insufficient resources for contracts covering anything more than emergencies and other urgent cases. The

DoH's 'draft guidance on capitation funding' (which, as described in Chapter 10, left many matters to the discretion of regional health authorities) presented the Region with an opportunity to strike back at what many believed to have been a cumulative 'overfunding' of practices. By the time the final version of the DoH guidance landed on their desk, regional officers had already begun to take action.

The Region commissioned outside help to develop a 'further refinement to the Department of Health approach'. This study looked at actual activity rates for fundholding hospital procedures by age and sex group in the Region as a whole, and applied these to data on activity rates by electoral ward in order to derive an 'actual to expected' ratio. It then tried to explain deviations from expected activity through regression analysis. After some experimentation, the researchers hit upon a combination of variables which appeared to explain a high proportion of the variation in activity rates. The variables were standardized mortality ratios for the population below 75, bed availability and unemployment as 'a proxy for socio-economic factors'.

The resulting formula had a very useful feature from the Region's point of view: had it been applied in 1992–3, it would have reduced by 20 per cent the capitation allocations in the county with the most practices, and it would have *increased* them in two areas with fewer fundholders. As a result, the formula allowed the Region to claim it had proved that this county's practices had been overfunded all along. They hoped that the findings of the study would exercise pressure on fundholding practices to accept lower budgets. What the study suggested, of course, was that in an area well endowed with hospitals and an articulate population, usage of hospitals was high. This is generally true; it is not confined to fundholders.

Regional officers were then given the task of explaining the study and its implications for budgets to the practices themselves. Talks with practices were conducted in an atmosphere affected by the leak of the story to the press and the rather violent reaction of some practices to the news, with threats to leave the scheme. Most practices accepted that budgets should be set in an equitable way, but contested the use of factors whose association with elective surgery was dubious.

In general, the Region's strategy appeared to be to try and 'claw back' from practices as much as it could get away with. For example, practices whose capitation-based targets were above their historic cost allocations would not have their budget increased unless they could prove 'the likelihood of real changes in justifiable workload'.

Budget setting was further complicated by 'erratic pricing'. Most hospitals in the Region had become NHS trusts, and clearly felt they could benefit from setting prices to fundholding practices high. Knowing that fundholding budgets had to take into account actual provider prices, many hospitals set different prices for fundholding practices, higher than those for districts. To justify this, hospitals argued that the two price sets were not comparable, as they applied to different types of contract, 'cost per case' and 'cost and volume' for practices, and 'block' for DHAs.

The controversy surrounding the regional formula and the problems with pricing delayed the process of setting the budgets. Eventually, many budgets were not set before May 1993 – two months into the financial year. Final budget allocations were affected by the attitude of the local FHSAs, who conducted the negotiations. It was agreed to move gradually towards the capitation formula suggested by the Region and to do more work on producing a fair allocation between fundholding and non-fundholding practices. In 1993–4, the hospital budgets in the disputed county were set near to the regional average for fundholders.

### Budget setting in the other regions

Region A had been much more successful in holding down budgets in the first two rounds. The 1992–3 hospital budgets in the region were £51 per patient, compared to £69 in Region B.

Budgets for the third wave were set on the basis of historic costs, using regional average activity rates as a yardstick. Region decided that practices whose historic costs were above the regional average would be awarded budgets on the basis of their historic costs, while those whose historic costs were below the regional average would be given budgets on the basis of the regional average. This was a much more generous approach.

As a result, hospital budgets to third-wave practices in Region A were as high as £70 per patient, compared to £53 for practices already in the scheme. Overall, total budgets per patient (excluding community health services) were up 18 per cent on the year before, from £102 to £121 per patient, despite the fact that per capita allocations to first- and second-wave practices in relation to the year before were raised by no more than 6 and 7 per cent respectively.

**Table 9.3** Fundholding budgets per patient in the three regions, 1993–4

| Region | Hospital (£) | Community (£) | Drugs (£) | Total (£) |
|---|---|---|---|---|
| A | 61.27 (13.54) | 7.67 (0.43) | 48.40 (11.60) | 128.23 (22.91) |
| B | 75.19 (12.62) | 19.09 (5.45) | 51.37 (8.23) | 155.89 (18.35) |
| C | 65.54 (10.87) | 18.57 (5.36) | 58.89 (9.04) | 154.49 (19.35) |
| All three RHAs | 68.97 (13.63) | 15.97 (6.88) | 52.61 (10.07) | 148.30 (22.69) |

The figures in parentheses are standard deviations.

Budget setting in Region C for the year 1993–4 was smooth and tough. Hospitals in the Region were using various pricing methodologies. One used a variant of the American diagnostic-related groups (DRGs) as part of a pilot programme that the Region aimed to implement in 1995–6. Another used the results of the Mersey costing exercise. Another used the BUPA pricing system, which it applied across all contracts and procedures, whether fundholding or not.

In contrast to the year before, when budgets to the second-wave practices (then joining the scheme) had been significantly higher than those to their first-wave colleagues, in 1993–4 allocations were more modest. First-wave practices saw their hospital allocations reduced from £62 per patient in 1992–3 to below £60 in 1993–4, while second-wave practices who had received £73 in the year before were only given £65. Third-wave practices were awarded just over £67 per patient for hospital care. Drugs budgets were in line with the regional average.

Overall, total budgets per patient (excluding community health services) were £136 per patient. First-wave practices were £128 (0.2 per cent up on the year before). Second-wavers were set at £139, reduced by 1.2 per cent. The third-wavers were awarded an average of £138 per patient. The rising trends of previous years had been checked (Table 9.3).

Budget allocations for all three years are shown in Table 9.4. The hospital budgets of the first-wave practices had been kept under close control. Subsequent waves were costing more.

**Table 9.4** Fundholding budgets in the three regions, 1991–2, 1992–3 and 1993–4

| | Patients | Funds | Budget allocations per capita (£) | | | |
| | | | Hospital | Drugs | Staff | Total |
|---|---|---|---|---|---|---|
| *1991–2* | | | | | | |
| 44 practices | 543,143 | 58,710,091 | 60.68 | 38.61 | 8.73 | 108.09 |
| *1992–3* | | | | | | |
| 44 first wave | 540,830 | 62,548,080 | 61.51 | 43.80 | 10.08 | 115.65 |
| 35 second wave | 386,642 | 47,616,720 | 65.50 | 46.80 | 10.64 | 123.15 |
| All 79 practices | 927,472 | 110,164,799 | 63.18 | 45.05 | 10.31 | 118.78 |
| *1993–4* | | | | | | |
| 44 first wave | 537,758 | 65,772,202 | 62.13 | 49.57 | 10.61 | 122.31 |
| 35 second wave | 382,719 | 49,875,810 | 68.08 | 51.43 | 10.81 | 130.32 |
| 107 third wave | 1,053,840 | 145,610,838 | 72.78 | 54.59 | 10.80 | 138.17 |
| All 186 practices | 1,974,317 | 261,258,851 | 68.97 | 52.61 | 10.75 | 132.33 |

'Total' in 1993–4 excludes community care.

# DISCUSSION

The entry of a large third wave of practices to the scheme in April 1993 intensified the basic issues. Historic cost budgeting allowed fundholding practices to benefit from a system that underwrites high referral rates. On top of this there was some suggestion from regions' analysis of what was happening that some trusts had begun to 'game' the system, trying to maximize revenue by charging fundholders higher prices than districts. They knew that fund-holders' budgets were set on the basis of local prices at the hospitals they used. In this situation it was only rational business practice to introduce a differential pricing strategy. The key to this perverse situation is that the discipline of the market, of which so much was made in the run-up to the reforms, is absent. A 'soft' budget constraint has been introduced for one set of purchasers.

The ultimate losers in this game are districts. Having ceded the direct management of most provider units in their jurisdiction, they have also relinquished any control over their pricing. The inflated GP budgets that may result are then taken away from districts' budgets.

The variety of the budgets set, illustrated in Table 9.5, is a reminder of the endemic and continuing inequity of resource allocation in general practice. Hospital budgets per patient in the 186 practices of the three regions examined here varied from £24 to £106, a ratio of 1 to 4.4. Total budgets ranged from £65 to £203 (1 to 3.1). The extent to which these variations correspond to underlying differences in the 'need' for health care of the registered population cannot be established with our current level of knowledge. However, it is hard to believe that these differences are large enough to warrant such a large variation in budget allocations between practices.

Furthermore, as seen before, per capita budgets in most areas were considerably increased with each additional wave of new practices, with the result that the later a practice joins the scheme the higher the budget it is likely to receive. Taking the three regions together, total budgets per patient in 1993–4 (excluding, for comparability, community health services) were on average £132 per patient, 11.4 per cent up on the year before, despite the fact that the first and second waves had their budgets increased by no more than 5.8 per cent. This points to a general pattern where once a high starting point is established for allocations to each new arrival to the scheme, budgets increase modestly thereafter.

**Table 9.5**   Third year practice budgets per capita (all prices in £s)

| Region B | Hospital | Community | Drugs | Staff | Budget | Excluding community health services |
|---|---|---|---|---|---|---|
| *1st wave* | | | | | | |
| 1 | 65.61 | 18.14 | 53.06 | 9.07 | 145.78 | 127.64 |
| 2 | 69.01 | 19.87 | 51.11 | 9.58 | 149.57 | 129.70 |
| 3 | 63.68 | 13.23 | 49.97 | 10.19 | 137.07 | 123.84 |
| 4 | 73.57 | 18.13 | 51.18 | 8.53 | 151.40 | 133.28 |
| 5 | 86.07 | 14.82 | 58.88 | 9.44 | 169.21 | 154.39 |
| 6 | 70.44 | 15.25 | 45.75 | 8.04 | 139.49 | 124.24 |
| 7 | 64.21 | 15.32 | 51.49 | 7.96 | 138.99 | 123.67 |
| 8 | 62.61 | 16.59 | 41.68 | 8.83 | 129.71 | 113.12 |
| 9 | 66.57 | 19.29 | 50.30 | 9.17 | 145.33 | 126.04 |
| 10 | 75.94 | 17.08 | 45.30 | 8.28 | 146.60 | 129.52 |
| 11 | 91.08 | 18.48 | 59.18 | 9.89 | 178.63 | 160.15 |
| 12 | 84.21 | 15.75 | 51.55 | 9.81 | 161.32 | 145.57 |
| 13 | 59.52 | 22.84 | 57.27 | 11.90 | 151.53 | 128.69 |
| 14 | 58.56 | 12.59 | 50.02 | 7.27 | 128.43 | 115.84 |
| 15 | 77.29 | 16.85 | 53.71 | 15.93 | 163.77 | 146.93 |
| 16 | 63.81 | 15.68 | 64.15 | 12.41 | 156.05 | 140.37 |
| 17 | 59.37 | 15.77 | 50.06 | 10.54 | 135.73 | 119.97 |
| 18 | 45.62 | 16.63 | 42.62 | 11.09 | 115.96 | 99.33 |
| 19 | 65.40 | 15.16 | 57.59 | 8.12 | 146.27 | 131.11 |
| 20 | 77.78 | 27.44 | 53.17 | 14.06 | 172.45 | 145.01 |
| 21 | 62.33 | 37.73 | 43.99 | 11.42 | 150.47 | 117.74 |
| 22 | 67.21 | 21.05 | 35.98 | 11.65 | 135.89 | 114.84 |
| *2nd wave* | | | | | | |
| 23 | 87.00 | 14.63 | 54.59 | 10.92 | 167.14 | 152.50 |
| 24 | 71.05 | 17.72 | 46.48 | 9.68 | 144.93 | 127.21 |
| 25 | 65.64 | 11.37 | 47.92 | 10.92 | 135.85 | 124.48 |
| 26 | 70.74 | 15.36 | 53.40 | 8.88 | 148.38 | 133.02 |
| 27 | 77.98 | 16.82 | 61.37 | 8.51 | 164.68 | 147.86 |
| 28 | 67.44 | 22.38 | 59.84 | 8.79 | 158.44 | 136.06 |
| 29 | 83.89 | 24.19 | 57.18 | 11.69 | 176.95 | 152.76 |
| 30 | 90.73 | 12.42 | 50.45 | 8.43 | 162.03 | 149.61 |
| 31 | 69.46 | 19.53 | 58.94 | 8.74 | 156.67 | 137.14 |
| 32 | 104.42 | 13.49 | 59.86 | 9.57 | 187.34 | 173.85 |
| 33 | 77.68 | 19.82 | 53.50 | 8.76 | 159.77 | 139.95 |
| 34 | 80.69 | 12.49 | 52.21 | 9.17 | 154.55 | 142.06 |

**Table 9.5** Continued

| Region B | Hospital | Community | Drugs | Staff | Budget | Excluding community health services |
|---|---|---|---|---|---|---|
| 35 | 69.11 | 36.55 | 47.56 | 8.90 | 162.12 | 125.57 |
| 36 | 71.78 | 17.05 | 30.92 | 10.78 | 130.53 | 113.47 |
| 37 | 63.37 | 20.31 | 51.84 | 16.72 | 152.24 | 131.93 |
| 38 | 56.38 | 17.99 | 37.30 | 11.96 | 123.63 | 105.64 |
| 39 | 66.51 | 23.18 | 57.94 | 11.19 | 158.81 | 135.63 |
| 40 | 82.93 | 16.14 | 38.18 | 14.54 | 151.80 | 135.66 |
| 41 | 55.52 | 15.12 | 40.28 | 15.00 | 125.91 | 110.79 |
| 42 | 61.98 | 14.72 | 33.65 | 9.03 | 119.39 | 104.66 |
| 43 | 79.02 | 20.31 | 37.22 | 13.51 | 150.06 | 129.75 |
| *3rd wave* | | | | | | |
| 44 | 67.73 | 20.78 | 55.05 | 8.53 | 152.09 | 131.31 |
| 45 | 80.94 | 22.73 | 64.51 | 12.43 | 180.61 | 157.88 |
| 46 | 73.38 | 18.53 | 48.72 | 10.71 | 151.33 | 132.80 |
| 47 | 70.53 | 16.63 | 59.39 | 9.50 | 156.05 | 139.42 |
| 48 | 76.36 | 16.03 | 53.23 | 9.60 | 155.22 | 139.19 |
| 49 | 70.86 | 23.35 | 44.10 | 9.70 | 148.00 | 124.65 |
| 50 | 83.44 | 19.99 | 58.57 | 8.78 | 170.68 | 150.69 |
| 51 | 62.01 | 20.10 | 52.89 | 8.93 | 143.94 | 123.84 |
| 52 | 70.73 | 16.49 | 44.72 | 8.83 | 140.77 | 124.27 |
| 53 | 75.38 | 12.87 | 49.94 | 10.34 | 148.51 | 135.64 |
| 54 | 79.33 | 18.66 | 49.58 | 9.13 | 156.71 | 138.05 |
| 55 | 71.89 | 19.93 | 58.55 | 9.14 | 159.50 | 139.58 |
| 56 | 79.68 | 13.00 | 44.80 | 11.22 | 148.70 | 135.70 |
| 57 | 83.39 | 17.99 | 45.79 | 8.42 | 155.59 | 137.60 |
| 58 | 75.77 | 15.06 | 56.11 | 9.29 | 156.23 | 141.17 |
| 59 | 75.55 | 20.86 | 54.88 | 9.55 | 160.84 | 139.98 |
| 60 | 84.40 | 21.53 | 46.34 | 12.69 | 154.96 | 143.43 |
| 61 | 77.91 | 16.57 | 57.16 | 11.29 | 162.92 | 146.35 |
| 62 | 101.06 | 21.70 | 45.35 | 8.05 | 176.16 | 154.46 |
| 63 | 75.52 | 18.94 | 62.97 | 8.32 | 165.75 | 146.81 |
| 64 | 54.26 | 17.56 | 51.13 | 12.27 | 135.23 | 117.66 |
| 65 | 79.42 | 17.22 | 56.10 | 9.40 | 162.14 | 144.92 |
| 66 | 86.47 | 35.16 | 60.88 | 9.58 | 192.08 | 156.92 |
| 67 | 72.93 | 30.02 | 64.63 | 10.09 | 177.67 | 147.66 |
| 68 | 57.43 | 24.60 | 60.93 | 5.87 | 148.82 | 124.22 |
| 69 | 75.13 | 25.61 | 59.70 | 7.94 | 168.38 | 142.77 |

**Table 9.5**   Continued

| Region B | Hospital | Community | Drugs | Staff | Budget | Excluding community health services |
|---|---|---|---|---|---|---|
| 70 | 68.78 | 14.57 | 45.78 | 12.27 | 141.40 | 126.83 |
| 71 | 92.33 | 32.47 | 59.21 | 6.65 | 190.66 | 158.19 |
| 72 | 97.49 | 22.30 | 44.02 | 12.26 | 176.07 | 153.77 |
| 73 | 81.28 | 20.88 | 55.35 | 15.94 | 173.46 | 152.58 |
| 74 | 64.65 | 15.25 | 29.45 | 12.67 | 122.02 | 106.77 |
| 75 | 74.19 | 24.05 | 62.92 | 16.58 | 177.74 | 153.69 |
| 76 | 67.18 | 19.65 | 48.92 | 10.60 | 146.35 | 126.70 |
| 77 | 103.33 | 24.07 | 48.97 | 9.44 | 185.81 | 161.74 |
| 78 | 98.56 | 24.91 | 66.17 | 13.09 | 202.72 | 177.82 |
| 79 | 68.07 | 24.20 | 48.92 | 9.32 | 150.51 | 126.31 |
| 80 | 89.24 | 30.96 | 65.42 | 12.05 | 197.67 | 166.71 |
| 81 | 81.87 | 26.22 | 53.67 | 12.17 | 173.93 | 147.71 |
| 82 | 91.42 | 17.11 | 48.56 | 12.52 | 169.61 | 152.50 |
| 83 | 96.77 | 21.58 | 38.84 | 11.77 | 168.96 | 147.38 |
| 84 | 105.59 | 24.50 | 46.08 | 10.75 | 186.92 | 162.42 |
| 85 | 59.91 | 9.85 | 38.82 | 9.04 | 117.61 | 107.76 |
| 86 | 88.41 | 15.64 | 35.41 | 11.30 | 150.75 | 135.11 |
| 87 | 105.06 | 9.50 | 45.55 | 8.53 | 168.64 | 159.14 |
| 88 | 71.16 | 29.04 | 54.14 | 12.66 | 167.00 | 137.96 |
| *All* | | | | | | |
| Average | 75.19 | 19.09 | 51.37 | 10.25 | 155.89 | 136.80 |
| Standard deviation | 12.62 | 5.45 | 8.23 | 2.19 | 18.35 | 16.09 |

The natural answer to the adverse efficiency and equity effects of historic cost budgeting revealed here seems to be a system of weighted capitation. The official position on the issue and the potential for successful solutions to the many policy problems it raises are discussed in more detail in the following chapters.

# 10

# INTRODUCING WEIGHTED CAPITATION

In Chapter 9 we described how regions actually went about the task of allocating fundholders a budget in the first three years of the scheme's existence. We saw that the method used essentially gave practices enough money to continue their referral rates and patterns at previous levels. Budgets then tended to grow incrementally. Yet this method of budget-setting totally destroyed the point of one of the original objectives of the scheme – to even out the apparently inexplicable variations in GP referral rates and to force GPs to think about the resource consequences of their decisions to refer patients to hospital (see Chapter 1). One of the things the reformers had objected to was that GPs could treat hospitals as if they were a free good. This tempted poor or lazy GPs to refer at sight rather than try to diagnose more carefully and treat themselves where possible. Historic cost incremental budget-setting defeated this purpose. Moreover, it rewarded high referral rates and it encouraged GPs to step up their referrals in the hope of increasing their budget.

To be fair, the DoH never wanted to go down this path, but had been forced to out of a combination of political expediency and administrative convenience. Official documents betray a gradual change of position as the Department, faced with the inherent difficulties of applying a formula funding approach, were driven to accept a historic cost basis for budget setting, at least temporarily. The consequences of the hurried original planning were coming home to roost.

## FROM CAPITATION TO HISTORIC COST BUDGETING

The 1989 White Paper had expressed what seemed to be an unequivocal commitment to capitation funding:

> Each practice's share will be based on the number of patients on its list, weighted for the same population characteristics as are proposed for allocations to districts. There are social and other local features which affect the use of hospital services, and these too will be reflected in the budget (Department of Health, 1989a).

Only later, in one of the more detailed Working Papers that followed the White Paper, did it appear that capitation funding was to be reserved for the future. The earlier commitment to it had now become vague:

> It is the Government's intention to move towards a weighted capitation approach to setting budgets in line with that proposed for RHAs and DHAs.

The document continued:

> Initially, however, budget setting will need to have regard to the different expenditure components contributing to the total budget. The hospital services component of the practice budget will be determined by comparison of the costs of the relevant services provided as a result of the practice's referral pattern in the previous year, with the average for the District(s), taking into account the number, age, sex and health of the practice's patients.

Still, a sort of compromise seemed to be envisaged:

> The actual budget will be set at a point between the two, taking account of local and social factors.

To underline this, a warning shot was fired:

> Budgets will not underwrite high referral rates for which there is no demonstrable cause (Department of Health, 1989b).

The reasons for this retreat are not difficult to deduce. First, the issues surrounding the construction of a weighted capitation formula were too complex to be resolved in the short time available.

Moreover, given the wide and seemingly inexplicable variations in referral patterns among practices, it was feared that capitation funding might damage the prospects of fundholding. As there was such a wide variation in GPs' use of hospitals any formula would be bound to strike a rough average usage rate. The high users would find they would have to cut their referral rates considerably. They would not join the scheme. The low users would gain a windfall, which would increase their demand for services and upset the Treasury. Signing-on as many eligible, willing and able practices as possible, soon became the political and hence managerial imperative for regional officers. The long-term dangers were evident. The DoH began to try to rescue the position.

## THE RETURN OF FORMULA FUNDING

Only a few months after the launch of fundholding, in August 1991, a working group on the funding of GP fundholders was set up, 'to make recommendations for introducing a capitation element to the budget setting methodology'. The membership of the working group was drawn from both the regional health authorities and the NHS management executive, district health authorities and FHSAs.

The work of the group initially concentrated on the hospital element of the budget. No change was thought to be necessary in the way the staff element of the budgets was set. On the other hand, a study to determine the factors that affect expenditure on drugs, commissioned from the University of Leeds, was discussed later when its results were available. The group submitted its interim recommendations, which were approved by the DoH and circulated for discussion to the regions in August 1992 in a document titled *Draft guidance on setting GP fundholder budgets in 1993–94*. The final version of that document was released in November 1992, as circular number (EL(92)83), outlining the official DoH policy to regional health authorities for budget setting in 1993–4.

In brief, the circular recommended no change to the methodology for setting the staff element of fundholding budgets. On the prescribing element of the budget, the document advised that in 1993–4 it should be set with reference on the one hand to historic costs and, on the other hand, to regional average costs per prescribing unit, adjusted for local factors.

Budget allocations for outpatient, community nursing and direct access services would continue to be based on historic cost. However, it was recommended that budget allocations for inpatient and day case services in 1993–4 should be set with reference to national average activity rates, adjusted for local factors, historic activity rates and actual local costs.

According to the DoH's guidance to regional health authorities, budget setting in 1993–4 should have aimed to provide equitable division of resources to all practices, whether fundholding or not. However, this aim was qualified with the following remark: 'The capitation-based benchmarks will not be sufficiently robust to act as the sole tool for budget setting in 1993–94 because of lack of data.' In view of this, the DoH advised that: 'Regions should determine the appropriate local pace of change in moving fundholder budgets towards capitation-based benchmarks.' The DoH document raises many issues. Before we discuss these, let us analyse the specific recommendations in more detail.

## HOSPITAL BUDGETS

The DoH working group examined separately the factors that might affect activity levels on one hand and treatment costs on the other. It was possible to look at average admission rates for each fundholding procedure, for example. Local factors might be found to explain variations in these rates, which would enable adjusters to be assigned that would vary by locality. Costs per procedure could be worked out at whatever level was appropriate – national, regional or FHSA. Activity rates and average costs for fundholding procedures, multiplied by one another, would eventually produce a weighted capitation allocation. This was the hope.

The working group examined the results of a study undertaken by Mersey RHA. The study, based on centrally available data, found no correlation between admission rates for elective surgery and standardized mortality ratios, unemployment rates, or the local supply of hospital beds. In view of this, the study recommended that only age and sex should be used as weights to determine the standard inpatient and day case admission rates to be incorporated in the formula.

In fact, the working group decided to pool the individual inpatient and day case procedures included in the scope of the

**Table 10.1** Fundholder procedure groups

| Speciality | Group | Examples of procedures |
|---|---|---|
| Ophthalmology | A | Laser for retinopathy, chalazion |
| | B | Cataract extraction, squint, glaucoma |
| ENT | A | Insertion of grommet, lesion of mucosa |
| | B | Laryngoscopy, adenoidectomy, pharyngoscopy |
| | C | Tonsillectomy, largyngectomy, tympanoplasty |
| Thoracic surgery | A | Bronchoscopy (day case) |
| | B | Bronchoscopy (inpatient), lung biopsy |
| | C | Balloon angioplasty – valvular and ischaemic |
| Surgery and urology | AA | Endoscopy, sterilization, varicose vein injection |
| | A | Hernias, varicose vein surgery, breast lesion |
| | B | Gall bladder, mastectomy, lithotripsy |
| | C | Gastrectomy, total or partial colectomy |
| Gynaecology | A | Colposcopy, hysteroscopy |
| | B | Sterilization, laparoscopy, vulval biopsy |
| | C | Ovarian cystectomy, hysterectomy |
| Orthopaedics | A | Ganglion, arthroscopy, trigger finger, bursa |
| | B | Hammer toe, tibial osteotomy, menisectomy |
| | C | Hip replacement, knee replacement, slip disc |

scheme, into a small number of 'fundholder procedure groups' at the subspeciality level. The 21 procedure groups were constructed so that each consisted of treatments with 'broadly similar costs'. Examples of procedures included in each group are given in Table 10.1.

National average activity rates for the fundholder procedure groups were drawn from the Hospital Expenditure Survey database. Results for 1989–90, the most recent year available, were

**Table 10.2**   Utilization rates, unit costs and costs per person by fundholder procedure groups – females

| Speciality | Group | Rate per 1000 | Unit cost | Cost per person |
|---|---|---|---|---|
| Ophthalmology | A | 0.47 | £580.02 | £0.27 |
|  | B | 3.12 | £871.23 | £2.71 |
| ENT | A | 1.31 | £582.63 | £0.76 |
|  | B | 1.04 | £679.82 | £0.71 |
|  | C | 2.06 | £737.46 | £1.52 |
| Thoracic surgery | A | 0.19 | £521.26 | £0.10 |
|  | B | 0.32 | £805.61 | £0.26 |
|  | C | 0.25 | £1425.75 | £0.35 |
| Surgery | AA | 11.90 | £601.04 | £7.15 |
|  | A | 8.24 | £645.47 | £5.32 |
|  | B | 1.70 | £1147.63 | £1.95 |
|  | C | 0.70 | £1879.09 | £1.31 |
| Urology | AA | 1.36 | £531.11 | £0.72 |
|  | A | 1.26 | £632.27 | £0.80 |
|  | B | 0.25 | £993.10 | £0.25 |
| Gynaecology | A | 8.34 | £332.04 | £2.77 |
|  | B | 4.59 | £381.69 | £1.75 |
|  | C | 4.23 | £1153.26 | £4.87 |
| Orthopaedics | A | 2.19 | £617.73 | £1.35 |
|  | B | 0.53 | £811.08 | £0.43 |
|  | C | 2.02 | £2111.08 | £4.27 |

applied and adjusted for 'under-reporting' to mirror better expected 1993–4 levels of activity.

On the other hand, the cost of inpatient and day case procedure groups was determined by splitting national average speciality costs into their fixed and variable cost components. More specifically, fixed costs are based on average speciality costs, while variable costs are based on procedure-specific average lengths of stay. Information from the same database was used. The NHS-specific hospital and community health services (HCHS) inflation index was applied to adjust costs to 1993–4 levels. The derived cost estimates corresponded to NHS 'revenue spending' only. No allowance for capital charges was made at this stage.

The resulting estimates of age- and sex-specific utilization rates for each fundholding procedure group, multiplied by their unit costs, could produce an approximation of the predicted cost per person of that age. If an average practice had 1000 male patients aged 25 to 55, it could expect to spend £$x$,000 per annum on hernia operations, for example. This might be spent by the district on non-fundholders or fundholders on their own patients. Therefore, a first estimate of the target-weighted capitation allocation to a practice can be given by adding the figures for age- and sex-specific cost per person across all procedure groups, and multiplying the sum by the number of patients in each patient group on the practice's list. There were 14 such groups, covering the age ranges 0–4, 5–14, 15–44, 45–64, 65–74, 75–84, and 85 and over for each sex.

The DoH national average estimates of inpatient and day case costs per procedure group are presented in Tables 10.2 and 10.3, for females and males, respectively. Only the average figure for all ages is shown, rather than the age-specific figures that are necessary for the application of the formula to the demographic profile of each practice's patient list.[1]

Nevertheless, limitations were introduced to the use of these capitation estimates. The DoH guidance clearly stipulated that, in view of the unreliability of data, actual provider prices rather than national average costs should remain the main consideration in budget setting:

> The main usefulness of the guideline speciality costs is in providing a comparator by which to assess the reasonableness of the prices being set in local provider units. Where significant variations are evident, Regions may wish to investigate the circumstances leading to these in the individual provider units.

The DoH guidance continued:

> However, fundholders should not be penalised simply because the local hospital has high prices: budgets should continue to be

[1] It is important to emphasize once more that the above method was applied to inpatient and day case procedures only. As regards outpatient services, due to the fact that admission data by age and sex were not available, the DoH recommended that regions should continue to rely on historic activity data at practice level and local provider prices.

**Table 10.3**   Utilization rates, unit costs and costs per person by
fundholder procedure groups – males

| Speciality | Group | Rate per 1000 | Unit cost | Cost per person |
|---|---|---|---|---|
| Ophthalmology | A | 0.44 | £521.30 | £0.23 |
| | B | 2.27 | £763.02 | £1.73 |
| ENT | A | 1.77 | £421.93 | £0.75 |
| | B | 1.56 | £521.31 | £0.81 |
| | C | 2.09 | £590.71 | £1.23 |
| Thoracic surgery | A | 0.41 | £448.20 | £0.18 |
| | B | 5.86 | £487.78 | £2.86 |
| | C | 0.76 | £1189.53 | £0.90 |
| Surgery | AA | 11.56 | £509.05 | £5.89 |
| | A | 6.96 | £659.26 | £4.59 |
| | B | 0.55 | £1109.82 | £0.61 |
| | C | 0.69 | £1641.99 | £1.13 |
| Urology | AA | 5.93 | £471.88 | £2.80 |
| | A | 3.80 | £590.12 | £2.24 |
| | B | 2.52 | £1013.63 | £2.56 |
| Gynaecology | A | 0.00 | £0.00 | £0.00 |
| | B | 0.00 | £0.00 | £0.00 |
| | C | 0.00 | £0.00 | £0.00 |
| Orthopaedics | A | 2.41 | £549.57 | £1.32 |
| | B | 0.70 | £609.67 | £0.43 |
| | C | 1.04 | £1679.13 | £1.75 |

set with reference to actual prices in 1993–94, pending greater
convergence of prices – at which time, national or local average
prices could be used in budget setting.

And, should any doubt still be left:

Regions are not required to take any account of these guidelines costs for budget setting, and may legitimately decide they
have no useful purpose locally.

Still, the introduction of local prices was only the first in a series of
adjustments regions would have to make to the capitation estimate.

The DoH recommended that the local significance of a list of factors should also be considered in determining the weighted capitation figure for each practice. These included:

- The proportion of a practice's patients with private health insurance.
- The number of referrals to Special Health Authorities and military hospitals, which are excluded from the NHS internal market.
- Local standardized mortality ratios, which may help predict the required number of cardiothoracic procedures.
- The current and planned split between inpatient and day case referrals.
- Local increases in activity rates since 1989–90, the last year for which data were available.

Furthermore, the DoH guidance assured regions that they would have 'full flexibility to take account of other important factors locally which they believe influence morbidity'.

Even after all the above adjustments have been made, the weighted capitation figure derived by the formula would still be only used as a 'benchmark' for budget setting.

## PRESCRIPTION BUDGETS

The Leeds University study of variations in prescribing costs had originally considered a series of factors (apart from age and sex), including premature mortality, low birth weight rates and self-reported permanent sickness and disability, on the basis of data collected by electoral ward. However, no clear pattern seemed to emerge from this analysis.

Subsequently, work towards the weighted capitation prescribing element of the budget concentrated on redefining the age and sex weighting of prescribing units as described in Chapter 7. The results of this study were reported in the *British Medical Journal*.

However, the DoH guidance proposed that limited use of these weightings should be made, in a manner similar to that for the hospital element of the budget. More specifically, it recommended that regional expenditure patterns in 1992–3 should be used as a starting point. These figures should be increased by 6.35 per cent to reflect the Treasury's estimate of increase in prescribing costs in

1993–4. Subsequently, the total amount of prescribing units in the region should be calculated on the basis of the age and sex structure of the region's population. This will produce a region-specific cost per prescribing unit, which, multiplied by the number of prescribing units corresponding to the practice's population, will provide the formula element of the prescribing 'benchmark'.

## REGIONAL VARIATION

The DoH had given wide latitude to regions in following its guidance on setting a formula. Regions duly differed.

Table 10.4 summarizes the way different regions approached the task and is taken from a survey undertaken by the journal *Fundholding*.

Nine of the English regions kept to a historic cost basis for setting budgets for 1993–4, though a number were hoping to move some way to incorporating a capitation formula in the negotiations in the next two years. Others were unconvinced of the need for anything but historic costs. At the other extreme Trent Region had used a form of capitation formula for the previous two years. North West Thames introduced its own version for 1993–4 and was seeking to move practices towards it over a period of years. Oxford was convinced of the need to move to a capitation-based allocation, not least to silence those complaining of the 'unfairly generous treatment of fundholders'. They were negotiating the basis for a formula with their fundholders.

## DISCUSSION

As the DoH put it, historic cost budgeting had 'contributed to the relatively smooth implementation of fundholding' but it could not be sustained in the longer run. Three arguments were put forward to support this view. According to the document, historic cost budgeting had been:

● *Inefficient*. 'Practices with traditionally low referring and prescribing rates are awarded lower budgets than high referrers and prescribers without any reference to relative need.'

**Table 10.4**    Region's use of the capitation formula for 1993–4

| Regions | Action |
| --- | --- |
| Northern | Historic activity costs only. Developing benchmarks but no date for use. |
| Yorkshire | Historic activity costs only. To include benchmarks in negotiations in 1994–5. |
| Trent | Elements of capitation used for past two years. District average treatment rates adjusted by age and sex factors. |
| East Anglia | Regionally adjusted national capitation formula used to alert region to high budgets and investigation. |
| NW Thames | Own version of capitation formula used. Aim to move practices towards these targets over a number of years. |
| NE Thames | Historic activity costs only. Capitation used for comparison by regional officers not for negotiation. |
| SW Thames | Historic activity costs for hospitals. Prescribing budgets to include capitation benchmark in the negotiations. |
| SE Thames | Historic activity costs. Next year hopes to use formula developed with fundholding. |
| Wessex | Historic activity costs. Capitation formula used to check results. Half above and half below what formula predicts. ASTRO PU used for drug budgets. |
| Oxford | Historic activity costs. Capitation used to check claims for special treatment. Aim to negotiate a formula with fundholders for next year. |
| Mersey | Historic activity costs basis. Used local benchmarks since first year in negotiations. |
| South Western | Historic activity costs rolled over unless 5% divergence. Capitation figures based on inpatient and day case surgery, outpatients the next year. Practices must argue hard to justify difference from formula. |
| West Midlands | Historic activity costs. Capitation figure given to practices for information. Used with some third-wavers in discussion on budget. |
| North Western | Historic activity costs. Capitation results to practices for information. |
| Scotland | Capitation benchmark used for inpatient and day case element. |
| Wales | Historic activity costs. Work on formula in 1993–4. |
| Northern Ireland | No work as yet. |

*Source: Fundholding*, 7 March 1993.

- *Inequitable*. 'No objective assessment of the appropriateness of the overall transfer of resources from DHAs to fundholders is made.'
- *Cumbersome*. 'As more practices become fundholders, the budget setting process needs to be stream-lined if it is to be administered efficiently.'

The DoH's view seems to us unanswerable. We saw in the previous chapter that, without a rigid formula basis, trust hospitals will push at the open door of GP fundholding budgets. The higher they set their prices the higher GP fundholders' budgets will be. As we argued at the beginning of this chapter, a formula is necessary to achieve the original efficiency goals of the scheme and without some common basis for allocating resources to fundholders and non-fundholders, the moral basis of the scheme will always be open to question.

To say this does not make the practical problem any easier to solve. Central to this is the fact that the variation in GPs' use of hospitals is so great. Any formula will therefore result in large numbers of losers for the reasons that were discussed at the beginning of the chapter. The variations between regional spending in 1976 were small by comparison and it took a decade to move regions near to their Resource Allocation Working Party formula targets. Districts are far from such a position after nearly 20 years.

Nevertheless, some features of the situation are more hopeful. If a national formula had been applied to first-wave fundholders in the early years of the scheme they would have received *more*, not less money, on average. Because they were relatively good practices, their historic cost budgets based on past referrals often tended to be lower than would have been produced by applying a national average formula to them. Oxford Region discovered that their fundholders had been 9 per cent underfunded in terms of the activity levels that applied to other GPs. Some other regions found the rates about the same. Nevertheless, there will be many losers, especially amongst some of the later cohorts and any move to a formula basis will take time. By the same token there will also be gainers, mostly practices in poorer, less demanding areas. The end result will be a more equitable allocation of resources between patients in different practices than has ever been achieved under the old system, but only so long as the same approach is applied to non-fundholding practices or the scheme is extended to cover all practices in some way. The main reason to believe that a move to formula funding is feasible is the restricted nature of the procedures the scheme covers. Fundholders are not like regions or districts. They are, at the moment, only responsible for non-emergency cases. Adjustments to new budget levels will affect the waiting patients, not life and death treatment. There is more scope for adaptation to new budget levels than some may suppose.

## Benchmarks versus targets

The concept of a 'benchmark' was introduced into the first guidance for the 1993–4 budgets. Although the word was reminiscent of the term 'targets' used in the RAWP resource allocation formula, in reality the analogy was only superficial. Some regions, it is true, interpreted their formula as a target towards which to move in a specified period. Others took the guidance more literally and merely used it as a background to the negotiations, waving it as a danger signal in front of high budget GPs. The term 'benchmark' encouraged this approach. The DoH was, it must be said, in a difficult position. The methodology of formula setting at this small practice level was poorly developed. The results of the 1991 Census were not then available. Any budgets set might change radically when new methods or data became available. It was difficult to demand that regions applied the guidelines in a rigid way. However, at some point soon, both method and data have to be improved to the point where benchmarks can become firm targets. 'Targets' should be the end point for convergence and stuck to even if progress towards them is slow. The DoH is working to that end. The expectation is that the formula basis can be developed further for 1995–6.

## Local prices

Regions were invited to substitute the prices of local hospitals for the national average costs listed in the appendix of the DoH guidance. National average costs were merely to be used to judge the 'appropriateness' of local pricing methods. Again the DoH was in a difficult position. Its aim was to get regions to move towards using average regional or national costs as quickly as possible, but the judgement was that this was not practicable in 1993–4. The aim is to move away from local pricing as quickly as possible.

However, in 1993 the incorporation of local prices into the budget-setting process gave hospitals the 'green light' to raise their prices during the course of budget negotiations, in the expectation that this would force regions to increase their allocations to practices and hence to the hospitals. This was self-defeating because the extra GPs' budgets came off district allocations and it introduced a new form of inequity between fundholders and non-fundholders.

Provider prices have failed to converge since 1991–2. In this respect, hospitals have been sheltered from the market discipline, which would, supposedly, produce a uniform pattern of prices in the NHS internal market. Faced with a soft budget constraint, the trust hospitals have exploited the situation. Evidence from one region in particular suggested that this was happening on a significant scale. The urgency of moving to a formula basis is clear.

**Other 'local factors'**

Apart from the incorporation of local provider prices, the local significance of a whole series of factors can also be included in determining the weighted capitation figure for each practice. Some of these factors are listed in the appendix of the DoH guidance, but regions are free to think of more. Again, according to the DoH, 'these factors could not have been included in the formula itself'.

But why not? The argument put forward in the guidance is that although some of these factors are common across the country, their local importance varies significantly. This is hardly convincing. Resource allocation formulae are general structures by design. Their real test is whether they are sensitive to those particular circumstances (e.g. region, district or practice) that are relevant for funding purposes. Resource allocations can then be decided by simply assigning to the variables in the formula values specific to the subject.

For example, had the Government intended to allow for the proportion of patients covered by private insurance, it could have set a capitation factor (e.g. equal to 0.5) for each privately insured patient, and coupled this with the requirement that participation in the scheme carried the responsibility for practices to disclose the number of private or privately-insured patients in their practice list. This would ensure a greater degree of fairness than currently prevails, and would enable fundholding practices to compete for patients with private insurance companies.

References to the incidence of very expensive patients and local morbidity levels raise the question of why the same factors were not listed as elements in the formula. The relationship between patient characteristics and the need for health care is exactly the issue the construction of a funding formula should be based upon. If they cannot be measured they should not be the basis for local nego-tiations. If they can be they should be in the formula.

The DoH is certainly on stronger ground in claiming that the task was simply too great to be accomplished for the 1993–4 guidance. Research has been commissioned from York University and the DoH is continuing to work on refining the formula.

While introducing local factors that cannot be avoided may be justified, the examples quoted in the guidance were unfortunate. Two examples are cited, the split between inpatient and day cases, and the increase in activity rates since 1989–90. If the DoH really wishes to encourage the wider use of day case treatments on the grounds of good practice and efficiency, it is absurd to penalize practices for doing just that, by reducing their budget allocations accordingly. As to budget adjustments following activity increases, we are back on historic cost territory: the more one refers, the more money one receives, irrespective of the underlying causes, which should have been identified and included in the funding formula.

**Bargaining**

The application of any funding formula is motivated by a desire to replace (or effectively reduce) bargaining by a more or less auto-matic mechanism of budget setting that is acceptable by all parties concerned. One of the attractions of such a mechanism is that it minimizes the administrative costs, and the inequity inherent in resource allocation by bargaining power.

It is clear from the description of the way the capitation formula is being used above that regions and FHSAs will continue to collect historic data at practice level in order to make decisions on actual budget allocations. In view of this, it is difficult to see how the DoH is hoping to achieve one of its main objectives, to 'stream-line' the budget-setting process in the interests of 'administrative efficiency'.

It has merely added another complexity. Furthermore, given that eventual allocations will be at an unknown point between historic costs and a 'capitation benchmark', the formula can at best be used to structure bargaining rather than replace it. The evidence clearly shows that practices bitterly contest regional attempts to reduce their allocation, especially when they doubt the validity of the underlying methods, and suspect them to be little more than a pretext, used by regions to 'claw back' what they believe is by rights theirs. This implies a return (if there ever was a departure) to 'rationing by decibels', a sadly familiar method of resource allocation, that allows little room for considerations of equity and efficiency.

**CONCLUSIONS**

From the discussion of the DoH guidance it appears that a common pattern can be detected. Faced with the difficult issues of resource allocation to fundholding practices, the DoH chose to relinquish its role as rule-maker and ultimate regulator of the NHS internal market. It let the regions decide if and how to determine what the 'right' budget for each practice should be, at least in the initial phases of the scheme. It was forced to do so because of the absence of adequate methodological work on formula-setting for small populations.

Improvements to the whole design of the capitation formula and its application are required. Ideally, a funding formula should link budget allocations to practices and to the characteristics of their patients alone. It should not interfere with variables that are endogenous to the system, such as referral habits, supply factors and local prices. Practices should be given a budget that reflects the average resource requirements for the treatment of their population in their region, and should be left alone to decide where and how to spend it in order to maximize patient welfare. Within a specified regulatory framework, nothing bar a change in the size and characteristics of the patient list should affect the following year's budget allocation.

As it is now, the capitation benchmark is not a benchmark at all. It is flawed by construction, loosely defined, and, therefore, open to manipulation. Moreover, it fails entirely to provide any indication of 'need', or the level of funding required as indicated by the characteristics of a practice's registered population. Finally, it allows the perpetuation of the inefficient and inequitable pattern of resource allocation in general practice, which fundholding has inherited from the pre-reform NHS.

In view of this, more work is urgently needed to identify the factors that should be incorporated into a weighted capitation formula to be used for setting fundholding budgets. This, however, raises the possibility of discrimination against individuals or entire patient groups who are potentially costly. What to do about this problem is discussed in Chapter 11.

# 11

# COUNTERING THE RISK OF BIASED SELECTION

In Chapter 10 we described how the DoH decided to return to the original intentions in the reforms and to move towards setting GPs' budget allocations using a weighted capitation formula. We also saw that the development of that formula is continuing. If it succeeds it will solve one set of problems but could open up another, notably the possibility of biased selection or choosing the cheap patient.

The possibility that patients might be refused registration with a fundholding practice has always been one of the most troubling concerns about the scheme. Observers from the United Kingdom (Crump *et al.*, 1991) and the United States (Weiner and Ferriss, 1990) had warned that biased selection might threaten the financial stability of the scheme. Scheffler (1989), having the experience of the American health maintenance organizations (HMOs) in mind, went so far as to suggest that biased selection might even prove to be the 'Achilles heel' of the NHS reforms.

## BIASED SELECTION IN PRE-PAID REMUNERATION SYSTEMS

The concept of biased selection has been explored extensively in the literature of the economics of imperfect information (Akerlof, 1970; Rothschild and Stiglitz, 1976). Biased selection in the specific case of medical care can take two forms: it can be initiated by the insurer or the insuree. Insurer-initiated biased selection may emerge where insurers receive a direct grant from the financing authority for every patient they agree to take on, according to the level of expenditure they are expected to generate. If insurers are in a position to predict the level of expenditure on each patient more accurately than the financing authority (a crucial assumption, as becomes clear later), they will be able to select those individuals whose levels of expenditure are expected to fall short of the grant or capitation income and refuse registration to all others.

As a result, an inadequate capitation formula provides insurers with an incentive to concentrate on attracting enrolees whose likely medical care expenditure is below that predicted by the formula, rather than to compete by designing more efficient methods of delivering services (Glennerster, 1992). This will create barriers in access to medical care, with some individuals finding it impossible to get insurance coverage. Evidence abounds that systems of pre-paid remuneration, such as the Medicare formula used to reimburse HMOs in the United States or the proposed system of payments to competing insurers in the Netherlands, leave substantial room for 'cream skimming' and discrimination against patients (Epstein and Cumella, 1988; van Vliet and van de Ven, 1990).

In the United Kingdom, as explained in Chapter 10, the capitation formula proposed by the DoH is only intended to help RHAs determine the inpatient element of fundholding budgets from the financial year 1993–4. However, we, and the DoH, have argued that a formula should be the basis for fundholding allocations in the long run. Will the existing DoH's formula be adequate for the task? In this chapter we will attempt to evaluate the performance of the formula from the point of view of incentives it might give for biased selection.

Naturally, it is too early for the actual impact of the new mixed method of capitation-informed funding to be analysed. For this reason, a simulation exercise was performed on the basis of data from 1991–2 using a sample of patients from a fundholding practice in England. Two crucial assumptions are made. The first is that the DoH formula is actually applied to determine the practice's final budget allocation. The second assumption is that the formula exactly predicts the total inpatient costs to the practice of services provided to the sample of patients. If it does not there will be scope for cream skimming.

## EMPIRICAL ANALYSIS OF PATIENT COSTS

As biased selection stems from the inadequate remuneration for patient-specific costs, it is necessary to examine the relationship between hospital expenditure in a fundholding practice and the known characteristics of its patients. Finally, we compare expected patient-specific costs as predicted on the one hand by our model using patient clinical histories available to the GP, and on the other hand by the DoH's formula, with actual costs in the practice under examination.

## Data

The actual cost of inpatient services charged to the practice by the provider on each occasion constitutes our first set of expenditure data. In order to construct this data set, financial reports for 1991–2 were collected on 1541 patients from a large fundholding practice, located in an ethnically and socially mixed area of a large town in England. The sample represented approximately 13 per cent of the total list of patients registered with the practice.

Next, the draft guidance of the DoH to RHAs was used to calculate the budget allocation the practice would receive for the sample. The 'capitation benchmark' has two main components: (1) average activity levels by age and sex for inpatient procedures covered by the scheme; and (2) average costs for fundholding procedures grouped according to severity and length of stay. The national average 'costs per person' (age- and sex-specific) presented in the appendix to the DoH draft guidance were entered into our database to estimate the budget allocation for a patient group with the demographic profile of the 1541 individuals in our sample. This gave us the budget the practice would have got for those patients if the present national formula had been applied adjusted to 1991–2 prices.

Finally, we used the past clinical experience of the patients to predict expenditure on them using the methodology presented in the next section. This gave us the expenditure the practice might have calculated it would incur for each class of patient using the information it had in its own records.

As our aim here is to analyse the extent to which the DoH formula provides incentives for 'cream skimming', it will be assumed that a practice intent on discriminating against expensive patients will try to make maximum use of information currently available to it. The most comprehensive source of such information is the patients' medical records.

**Table 11.1** Predictors of inpatient expenditure

|  | *Mean* | *Definition* |
|---|---|---|
| *Variable* |  |  |
| Age | 40.6 | As of April 1992 |
| Sex | 0.497 | Male = 0; female = 1 |
| Deprivation | 0.234 | Medium = 2; low = 1 (77 no records) |
| Smoking | 0.326 | No = 0; yes = 1 (1053 no records) |
| Hypertension | 0.195 | Threshold: 140 mmHg systolic, 90 mmHg diastolic No = 0; yes = 1 (667 no records) |
| *Diagnostic groups: no = 0, yes = 1 (examples of conditions included)* |  |  |
| Cancer | 0.019 | e.g. mastectomy, hysterectomy (if cancer-related) when patient of child-bearing age (below 45 years) |
| Heart/stroke | 0.133 | e.g. angina, ischaemic heart disease, cardiac catheter, myocardial infraction, meningitis, coronary artery disease |
| Stomach/liver | 0.060 | e.g. gall bladder, duodenal or stomach ulcer, colitis, oesophageal reflux, pyloric stenosis, gastrectomy |
| Kidney | 0.031 | e.g. renal failure, nephritis, pyeloplasty/hydronephrosis, haematuria, intravenous pyelogram |
| Lungs | 0.113 | e.g. asthma, chronic bronchitis, bronchospasms, haemoptysis, tuberculosis, pertussis (if child) |
| Spine | 0.211 | e.g. arthritis, haemarthrosis, osteoarthritis, rheumatism, arthrosis, spinal infections, displacement of intervertebral disc, lumbar, arthrodesis, cervical rib, scoliosis |
| Minor surgery | 0.154 | e.g. varicose veins, hernia, haemorrhoids, cataract |
| Disability | 0.013 | e.g. spina bifida, polio, paraplegic hemiparesis, paralysis, cerebral palsy |
| Mental disorder | 0.106 | e.g. depression, schizophrenia, neurosis, suicidal, alcohol abuse, drug abuse |
| Diabetes | 0.024 | diabetes mellitus |

The medical records, in addition to the demographic profile of patients, summarize the doctor's knowledge of their medical history. The medical notes list medication regime, episodes of hospitalization, diagnostic details and follow-up assessments from GP consultations. From the medical records, 16 explanatory variables were produced, reflecting socio-demographic, behavioural and diagnostic factors. The methodology of variable construction is fully reported elsewhere (Matsaganis and Glennerster 1994). For a brief description of the explanatory variables see Table 11.1.

### Skewed spending

The first results confirmed the kind of picture Scheffler (1989) and others had predicted.

The distribution of expenditure on the limited range of inpatient procedures covered by fundholding was extremely skewed. As Table 11.2 shows, only 69 patients (4.5 per cent of the sample) incurred any expenditure for inpatient services at all. One patient accounted for 10 per cent of all costs for these services, while 1 per cent of patients required 44 per cent of total inpatient expenditure.

**Table 11.2**  Cumulative distribution of inpatient expenditure

| Highest-cost patients | Cost (£) | Percentage of total cost |
|---|---|---|
| 1 patient | 4,824 | 9.9 |
| Top 1% (15 patients) | 21,588 | 44.2 |
| Top 4.5% (69 patients) | 48,804 | 100.0 |

The non-normal distribution of the dependent variables made the estimation of determinants of expenditure by ordinary least squares (OLS) inappropriate. In order to diminish the influence of extreme values, a logarithmic transformation of total hospital costs was used. Furthermore, in order to deal with the considerable skewness of the distribution of hospital expenditure, a two-part model was applied. In other words, the probability of patients using the relevant hospital services was determined first, followed by the estimation of the expected level of hospital expenditure, conditional on it being positive.

Readers who wish to avoid the mathematics may skip the next section.

## The model

Let us define the expected level of inpatient expenditure $(Y)$ dependent on a vector of explanatory variables $(X)$ as:

$$E(Y \mid X)$$

The probability $P_i$ of positive medical costs for a patient with characteristics $X_i$ is:

$$P_i(Y_i > 0 \mid X_i)$$

The individual probabilities of positive medical costs can be calculated from a logit equation for the full sample of patients:

$$I = \alpha + \beta X + \epsilon$$

The errors $\epsilon$ are distributed as $N(0,1)$. As:

$$I_i = \log_e(P_i/(1 - P_i))$$

it follows that:

$$P_i = e^{I_i}/(1 + e^{I_i})$$

Once the individual probabilities have been computed, a linear model on the logarithmic scale can be estimated by OLS for patients with positive expenditure only:

$$\log(Y \mid Y > 0) = \gamma + \delta X + \eta$$

The errors $\eta$ are distributed as $N(0,\sigma^2)$.

Expected expenditure $E(Y \mid X)$ for the $i$ individual is calculated as:

$$E(Y_i \mid X_i) = P_i \cdot Z_i \cdot \phi$$

$Z_i$ is the logarithmic retransformation of the estimates of $\log (Y_i \mid Y_i > 0)$, and $\phi$ denotes the retransformation factor needed to correct for the residuals $\eta$ in the OLS equation (Duan *et al.*, 1983).

## Results

Overall closeness of fit in qualitative models can be measured by Effron's $R^2$ (Maddala, 1988), based on the sum of squared differences between observed and expected values. More specifically, in models of medical expenditure where expected values are obtained from a two-part process, Effron's $R^2$ can be used as an acceptable measure of overall explanatory power (Newhouse *et al.*, 1989).

Effron's $R^2$ for the predicted values estimated from the model of patient characteristics was found to be 3.43 per cent (3.42 per cent unadjusted for budget neutrality), while for the predicted values obtained directly from the DoH formula it was calculated to be 1.46 per cent (1.30 per cent unadjusted for budget neutrality).

From the point of view of closeness of fit, these results are rather disappointing. Nevertheless, low $R^2$s are not uncommon in the literature of determinants of health expenditure. In the United States, several studies have shown that the Medicare formula can explain only about 1 per cent of the total variation in costs incurred by elderly HMO enrolees (Lubitz *et al.*, 1985; Epstein and Cumella, 1988). In the Netherlands, van Vliet and van de Ven (1990) found that a similar formula proposed for the reimbursement of private insurers explained 2.4 per cent of the total cost variation. The reason for this failure is simply that a great part of the variance in medical costs is not related to known patient characteristics. In other words, it is impossible to predict.

The phenomenon of 'regression towards the mean' is a reflection of this. Welch (1985) showed that if a sufficiently large group of patients with medical expenditures $100 above average is selected, their subsequent expenditures are likely to be $20 above average in the first year, $16 in the second year, and $13 in the third year. The extent to which medical expenditures average out over time indicates the random component of the variance. Conversely, the degree to which expenditures persist at above average levels shows the systematic part of the variance. This is attributed to patient-specific factors that are constant over time, e.g. their chronic health status. In the light of regression towards the mean, Welch (1985) suggested that 'one can explain no more than 20 per cent of the variance in such equations'. In fact, empirical studies in the United States and the Netherlands have put the maximum explainable variance at around 14 per cent (Newhouse *et al.*, 1989; van Vliet and van de Ven, 1990).

The fact that the distribution of medical expenditure is predominantly random implies that the maximum achievable predictive power of models intended to explain it will inevitably be low. In view of this, the adequacy of a capitation formula should be judged in comparison to realistic alternatives rather than in absolute terms.

**Table 11.3** Sex and age distribution of inpatient expenditure – females

| Age group | Number of patients in group | Average cost per patient | | Actual |
|---|---|---|---|---|
| | | Predicted | | |
| | | Model | Formula | |
| <4 | 41 | £19.07 | £8.23 | £18.98 |
| 5–14 | 60 | £28.37 | £10.18 | £0.00 |
| 15–24 | 103 | £8.67 | £25.44 | £8.33 |
| 25–34 | 134 | £17.34 | £25.44 | £29.31 |
| 35–44 | 92 | £49.46 | £25.44 | £98.74 |
| 45–54 | 91 | £19.14 | £39.46 | £14.79 |
| 55–64 | 87 | £30.29 | £39.46 | £30.98 |
| 65–74 | 74 | £99.79 | £52.77 | £63.39 |
| 75–84 | 66 | £95.43 | £69.83 | £0.00 |
| >85 | 18 | £104.36 | £71.33 | £238.44 |
| All females | 766 | £39.41 | £34.13 | £36.13 |

If a practice, even using a sophisticated model, cannot predict which kinds of patient are going to be expensive that is good news from the point of view of cream skimming. Cream skimming will arise therefore, not as a result of the low predictive power of the formula alone, but because of the ability of insurers (fundholding practices in our case) to better predict the costs of defined patient groups than the formula. Therefore, the success of a capitation formula in narrowing the scope for discrimination against patients depends on the magnitude and the direction of the prediction errors for definable groups of patients, rather than on overall predictive power as indicated by $R^2$s.

In short, was our formula, which represents a fictional ruthless practice's best efforts, better able to predict the cost of its patients than the DoH's formula? The answer, unfortunately, is yes.

It is necessary for our analysis to compare expected expenditure $E(Y_i)$ to actual expenditure $Y_i$ *for individuals with certain common characteristics*, as implied by $X_i$. In order to evaluate the performance of the DoH funding formula compared to that of our model, predicted costs from both are examined alongside the actual costs for certain patient groups. Tables 11.3 and 11.4 compare these

**Table 11.4**   Sex and age distribution of inpatient expenditure – males

| Age group | Number of patients in group | Average cost per patient | | |
|---|---|---|---|---|
| | | Predicted | | Actual |
| | | Model | Formula | |
| <4 | 39 | £10.47 | £16.13 | £9.56 |
| 5–14 | 64 | £17.08 | £11.55 | £31.48 |
| 15–24 | 99 | £4.65 | £12.77 | £4.02 |
| 25–34 | 148 | £10.51 | £12.77 | £4.16 |
| 35–44 | 116 | £27.98 | £12.77 | £14.77 |
| 45–54 | 93 | £11.24 | £32.55 | £14.61 |
| 55–64 | 83 | £20.30 | £32.55 | £12.09 |
| 65–74 | 83 | £69.08 | £71.44 | £90.82 |
| 75–84 | 44 | £65.57 | £100.37 | £128.20 |
| >85 | 6 | £83.50 | £97.10 | £79.33 |
| All males | 775 | £24.02 | £29.24 | £27.27 |

estimates for patient groups defined by age and sex, while Table 11.5 presents actual and expected costs for patient groups defined on the basis of other individual characteristics from the medical records.

## THE SCOPE FOR BIASED SELECTION IN FUNDHOLDING

It can be assumed that the 'intelligence' required to engage in biased selection by fundholders would be limited to the information found in the medical records. This is particularly true in the short term. In the long term, practices will be able to collect data on the previous costs, as well as on the chronic health of an individual patient, if they so choose. Therefore, our model, which replicates the kind of information a practice could gain, can be used to estimate the maximum scope for cream skimming allowed by the DoH formula.

The opportunities for manipulating a capitation formula adjusted for age and sex by using information on further determinants of expenditure can be illustrated with some examples.

**Table 11.5** Distribution of inpatient expenditure – patient groups

| Patient group | Number of patients in group | Average cost per patient | | Actual |
|---|---|---|---|---|
| | | Predicted | | |
| | | Model | Formula | |
| Clean record | 703 | £18.84 | £23.25 | £15.55 |
| Diabetes | 37 | £102.46 | £46.77 | £90.92 |
| Cancer | 28 | £39.98 | £51.27 | £43.57 |
| Heart/stroke | 205 | £61.52 | £50.09 | £66.47 |
| Stomach/liver | 94 | £36.27 | £41.61 | £33.45 |
| Kidney | 48 | £85.36 | £43.69 | £77.91 |
| Lungs | 173 | £26.04 | £32.90 | £45.41 |
| Spine | 326 | £37.14 | £44.74 | £32.81 |
| Minor surgery | 238 | £79.79 | £45.10 | £74.52 |
| Disability | 19 | £72.12 | £39.56 | £56.47 |
| Mental disorder | 164 | £41.39 | £34.67 | £63.39 |
| Moderate deprivation | 97 | £41.51 | £36.52 | £38.13 |
| Smoking | 159 | £25.39 | £29.71 | £60.82 |
| Hypertension | 170 | £59.05 | £54.00 | £65.14 |
| All patients | 1541 | £31.67 | £31.67 | £31.67 |
| $R^2$ | | 3.43% | 1.46% | |

Consider the case of the 37 patients suffering from diabetes. If an RHA used the DoH formula alone to set the budget of a fundholding practice the situation might be as follows. As Table 11.5 implies, the practice would be offered £1730 towards the cost of inpatient services for these patients (that is, the average formula allocation of £46.77 per patient, multiplied by 37). By definition, this is equal to the allocation for an equal number of non-diabetics with identical demographic characteristics. A quick check with the medical records would show that these patients, far from 'average', actually suffered from diabetes. The practice would then identify these patients as likely to cost considerably more than the formula had allowed.

If the practice had access to a predictive model like the one used here, expected expenditure on the 37 diabetes patients would be estimated at £3791 (that is, £102.46 multiplied by 37). Alternatively, the practice could search the financial records of previous years in order to find out the past costs of the group of 37 diabetics. In 1991–2 these patients actually cost the fundholding practice examined here £3364 (from Table 11.5, £90.92 times 37).

It is therefore clear that a small number of patients could cost the practice roughly between £1600 and £2000 in extra, non-reimbursed, inpatient expenditure. Considering that our sample represents only one-eighth of the practice's patient list, by implication the potential financial gains from a discriminating strategy against a single patient group could be tens of thousands of pounds.

The case of diabetes sufferers is not untypical in the sample examined here. In general, Table 11.5 indicates that the DoH formula would systematically underestimate the actual cost of inpatient services to the practice for most of the patient groups identified in the table. Invariably, our model of predictors extracted from medical records produced more accurate estimates of average costs than the DoH model.

Conversely, let us focus on the 703 patients in the sample whose medical records contain nothing but their name, age and address – in other words, patients with a 'clean' record, who presumably enjoy good health. In contrast to the previous example, the DoH formula would overestimate the practice's average expected inpatient expenditure by between £7.70 (compared to actual costs in the first year of the scheme) and £4.41 (compared to costs predicted on the basis of our model). A fundholding practice with the intention to cream-skim could actively seek to attract such financially desirable patients. Considering that healthy individuals are by far the largest group in the patient list of any practice, the incentive to do just that is not negligible.

The cost of hospital services as a whole (in other words, both inpatient and outpatient) would seem to be a more reasonable choice for a funding formula because the frequency of positive values is greater and the skewness of the distribution less pronounced than is the case with inpatient costs alone. However, the DoH working party considered but rejected (on the grounds of low accuracy and availability of data) the inclusion of outpatient costs in the computation of 'capitation benchmarks'.

In order to provide a comparable estimate of formula allocations for the reimbursement of total hospital costs, the two-part model of predictors from the medical records was re-estimated with the sum of inpatient and outpatient costs as the dependent variable, alongside a similar model with age and sex as its only predictors (intended

**Table 11.6** Distribution of total hospital expenditure – patient groups

| Patient group | Number of patients in group | Average cost per patient | | Actual |
|---|---|---|---|---|
| | | Predicted | | |
| | | Model | Age and sex | |
| Clean record | 703 | £45.17 | £31.15 | £29.49 |
| Diabetes | 37 | £163.10 | £73.98 | £153.63 |
| Cancer | 28 | £168.79 | £88.94 | £121.92 |
| Heart/stroke | 205 | £104.70 | £76.31 | £112.22 |
| Stomach/liver | 94 | £81.16 | £66.86 | £76.19 |
| Kidney | 48 | £111.30 | £68.38 | £133.92 |
| Lungs | 173 | £73.05 | £55.40 | £72.61 |
| Spine | 326 | £81.17 | £71.92 | £70.18 |
| Minor surgery | 238 | £94.41 | £70.99 | £112.80 |
| Disability | 19 | £99.58 | £62.80 | £82.97 |
| Mental disorder | 164 | £88.18 | £59.51 | £117.75 |
| Moderate deprivation | 97 | £66.42 | £60.34 | £65.07 |
| Smoking | 159 | £56.12 | £52.55 | £89.55 |
| Hypertension | 170 | £84.48 | £83.15 | £106.80 |
| All patients | 1541 | £55.50 | £55.42 | £56.71 |
| $R^2$ | | 3.86% | 1.72% | |

to simulate the effects of the DoH formula). The results, fully discussed elsewhere (Matsaganis and Glennerster, 1994), are presented in Table 11.6. It can be seen that the comprehensive model performed better than with inpatient costs only as the dependent variable, whether its predictions are compared to those of the age and sex model, or to the actual costs incurred by the practice.

## IS CREAM SKIMMING A REAL THREAT IN FUNDHOLDING?

The findings of our study, in common with those overseas studies of biased selection mentioned earlier, show that cream skimming in the specific context of fundholding is both technically feasible and financially profitable.

It is undeniable that the ethics of general practice in the United Kingdom, reinforced by the founding principles of the NHS at work, are a powerful defence against cream skimming. Our GPs were appalled at the suggestion that they would ever do such a thing. If fundholders were suspected of it they might well lose custom. However, reliance on medical ethics alone would be ill-advised, as American experience shows us. Newhouse (1982) has noted that Blue Cross plans in the United States had maintained a policy of 'community rating' until commercial insurance health carriers entered the market offering 'experience rating', which threatened Blue Cross' market share, and forced Blue Cross plans to follow suit.

Administrative measures against cream skimming are equally bound to provide only a short-term solution. If biased selection does become worth while, strategies aimed at encouraging good risks to join the practice and bad risks to leave are certain gradually to become too subtle to be detected by the authorities that will be given the task of monitoring the situation. The personal nature of the doctor–patient relationship makes it relatively easy for doctors to persuade financially unattractive patients that it is in their own interest to seek medical care elsewhere (Newhouse, 1982).

The likely failure of medical ethics or administrative regulations to prevent cream skimming other than in the short term leaves adjustments to the capitation formula as the only viable alternative.

## FORMULA ADJUSTMENTS AGAINST CREAM SKIMMING

How should the formula be revised and is it practicable? Both in the United States and the Netherlands, although there is broad agreement that demographic factors are poor predictors of future medical expenses, there is also recognition of the shortcomings of prior costs or utilization on one hand, and health status on the other, as potential candidates for inclusion in a capitation formula.

The use of individual past costs in budget setting is likely to remove incentives to cream skimming, but has other perverse effects. It would encourage doctors to use expensive treatments with certain groups of patient. Practical considerations, such as the unavailability of data on past expenses incurred by new entrants to the system, are also powerful arguments against reliance on prior costs as a measure against cream skimming.

On the other hand, there is concern that chronic health indicators could be open to manipulation not dissimilar to the phenomenon of 'DRG creep' in the United States (the reclassification of borderline diagnostic cases in order to maximize reimbursement revenue; Newhouse, 1986; Howland *et al.*, 1987; Epstein and Cumella, 1988; Ash *et al.*, 1989; Newhouse *et al.*, 1989). Diagnostic Related Groups (DRGs) are categories of treatment used to define costs and reimbursements for private insurance. Hospitals tend to define illnesses in higher cost and reimbursement categories than clinically justified in order to maximize their revenue. In view of this, the introduction of chronic health adjusters to the DoH formula in the United Kingdom would require careful design and reasonable monitoring arrangements. However, the results of our study indicate that the ability of a modified formula to eliminate incentives for cream skimming could be improved significantly. Such a formula need not, and cannot, predict spending accurately. It merely has to be able to do as well as, or better than, an individual GP could.

Furthermore, it is likely that the collection of the necessary data would coincide with the introduction of health promotion initiatives in primary care that provide practices with financial incentives to assemble databases on the morbidity of their registered population. It would be possible to set perhaps no more than eight or ten indicators of prior treatment or chronic status that would attract an enhanced budget allocation. These indicators might look very like our variables. Practices would have an incentive to inform FHSAs about patients who fell in these at-risk categories and hence receive more funding. Just as income tax claims are not all checked in detail every time, the practices would merely have to be able to produce proof for a sample audit trail. The penalties for incorrect claims could be very severe. Again it must be noted that the British problem is manageable just because fundholding only deals with a small range of less expensive procedures, unlike the situation in the United States or the Netherlands.

A whole range of elaborations to the formula solution have been proposed in the United States (for example, Luft, 1986; Newhouse, 1986; Howland *et al.*, 1987; Wallack *et al.*, 1988; Newhouse *et al.*, 1989), but they are unnecessary in the United Kingdom. Robinson *et al.* (1991), for example, suggested that outlier cases could be reimbursed on a fee-for-service basis rather than through a formula. In fact, this already happens in the fundholding scheme (the £5000 ceiling and the exclusion of very expensive procedures). Our problem is less daunting.


## CONCLUSION

Biased selection is not yet a major worry. It is likely, moreover, that this will remain so even after the introduction of an element of formula funding in budget setting. Nevertheless, we have shown that the future application of a capitation formula based on the DoH guidelines is certain to introduce incentives for cream skimming.

In the short term, these incentives will be dealt with in one of two possible ways. On one hand, the DoH will probably retain elements of negotiation and historic cost arguments in budget setting. On the other hand, costs may be shifted to practices who happen to have a higher than average proportion of expensive patients on their lists. Both outcomes are undesirable; the former for perpetuating the inefficiency and inequity of the previous system of budget setting, and the latter for preparing the psychological ground for biased selection in the not too distant future.

Our study has demonstrated that it *is* possible to benefit from the incentive advantages associated with capitation funding, without at the same time giving hostages to fortune in the form of incentives for discriminatory behaviour against certain patient groups. Our analysis showed that the potential benefits in terms of reducing the opportunities for cream skimming can be quite considerable. It is therefore important that the Government consider the possibility of using chronic health status adjusters to improve the capitation formula. The DoH was, in fact, planning to do this in 1994.

# 12

# THE BALANCE SHEET

We began this study by remarking that GP fundholding provided, in microcosm, a test case for the new-style competitive welfare society. In this final chapter we review the arguments and look at the balance sheet.

## THE CASE AGAINST STATIST WELFARE

The economic crises of the 1970s and the Conservative Governments of the 1980s shook the traditional welfare state to its foundations. The check to economic growth caused both the Labour and the Conservative Governments of the period to halt the steady incremental growth of state spending on social policy as a share of national production that had gone on for most of the century (Hills, 1993). This was nowhere more important than in the case of the NHS. In the two decades before 1976, NHS expenditure had risen annually at twice the rate of the national income. In the early 1980s spending on the NHS was to rise only half as fast as the national income and more slowly than the demands of an increasingly elderly population (Owens and Glennerster, 1990). This put increasing pressure on the service and caused political embarrassment as waiting lists grew. Shortages of resources were not the only factor at work, however. Monopolistic forms of provision and the weak position of consumers and patients began to put the services at increasing political disadvantage in a consumerist world. The Conservative reforms, therefore, had two main objectives:

1  To get more health care from the limited budget the Government was prepared to provide.
2  To increase the responsiveness of the NHS to consumers.

These objectives were not exactly the same, or even entirely compatible. This was reflected in the debates that took place within the Government and on the review group. They were consequently reflected in the reform package that emerged (Thatcher, 1993). There was a common thread – the separation of purchasers of health care from providers, like hospitals This was intended to introduce an element of competition, which would put hospitals on their toes. In trying to get purchasers' custom they would improve the quality and cost of their activities.

One model of reform, that in which the district health authority became the monopoly purchaser, was essentially concerned to improve the efficiency of the hospital unit and to improve planning. It was not well adapted, by its very nature, to be responsive to consumers. Indeed, by only contracting with a smaller range of hospitals this model tended to restrict GPs' freedom to refer where they wanted, or so GPs feared. Patients had no choice of purchaser.

The GP fundholding model embodied a quite different principle. Patients should be able to choose between those who would purchase services on their behalf, in this case GPs. Competition would be introduced on *both* the purchasing and the providing side of the market. Here too, there were problems. The nearest example of this model at work were the American Health Maintenance Organizations (HMOs). But they were much larger than any British GP practice, and the smaller ones were subject to budget instability. They also had a tendency to exclude less healthy, more costly patients in the competition to stay viable. The fundholding scheme, described in Chapter 2, was designed to avoid these problems. Only large practices could join and, by concentrating on non-emergency, outpatient and pathology services, and restricting the scheme to patient costs below £5000, it was hoped to avoid the budget volatility problem. The areas targeted for GP purchasing were however, arguably the most inefficient parts of the NHS for reasons we discussed in Chapters 1 and 6.

The British health reforms, therefore, went ahead combining two very different models of purchasing – district- and GP-based. This study has compared the advantages and disadvantages of both.

## IMPLEMENTING THE SCHEME

Early reactions to the reforms suggested that giving budgets to GPs would be impracticable. It was indeed true that this part of the reforms was only sketched in outline in the White Paper. In fact, the DoH and the regional officers involved did a remarkable job in getting the scheme off the ground, as we described in Chapter 4. It proved far more popular than many of those involved thought it would be. Many of the early GP joiners were concerned to preserve their freedom to refer patients and saw fundholding as a way of doing that. They also wanted to increase the leverage they had over hospitals to improve services, and this motive became more and more important as the study progressed. Third-wavers saw that first-wavers had succeeded in making hospitals take note and respond to their complaints, a shift in the balance of power back to general practice for the first time this century.

As we saw in Chapter 1, health care markets are not like the idealized simple market place. Purchasers are at a severe disadvantage compared to health care providers in the information they have at their disposal. We found this particularly true of districts in making detailed contract specifications. We compared the contracting done by GPs and districts to see how far they had been able to improve the efficiency of the system.

## THE EFFICIENCY CRITERION

### Hospital efficiency

Even if every GP were a fundholder, less than one-fifth of hospital expenditure would be purchased by them. Thus their impact on hospitals for good or ill is likely to be limited. However, their purchasing power was concentrated on those parts of the hospital service that has performed least well over the years – elective surgery waiting times, pathology and outpatient care.

The evidence we presented in Chapter 6 on the way fundholders have used their market power suggests to us that this model of contracting is working in very much the way the reformers had in mind. GPs have had the motivation and the information to seek better contracts. They have been able to diversify their providers, bringing to bear a real threat of exit, and provide their patients with choice and speedier and better service. This has been achieved for the most part by switching to more effective providers or by improving the performance of the same provider.

A competing system of decentralized purchasing has forced districts to improve their contracting skills and to invent new ways of involving GPs in their contracting process. GPs, being closer to the pains and preferences of patients, have been more likely to reflect these in their contracts.

In short, the original Maynard hypothesis, outlined in Chapter 1, does find support in our study of the contracting process since 1991. It was confirmed by our interviews with intending third-wave practices, who gave as their main reason for joining the scheme the impact they saw first-wavers had had on local hospitals. Howie's (1993) assessment of the Scottish experience reaches a similar conclusion.

Medical researchers may, understandably, like harder evidence. Are patients more healthy as a result? The problem is that we cannot readily apply randomized control trial methods to this kind of question. The very hypothesis from which the contestable market theory begins is that every actor will be affected by the introduction of a competitive environment not just fundholders. Once the pathology monopoly was broken it affected non-fundholders as well as fundholders.

**Allocative efficiency between sectors**

The second hypothesis was that combining primary and secondary care budgets would enable services to shift to the most convenient site. The removal of budget boundary walls between hospital, practice and community services *has* begun to produce more flexibility and a growth in practice-based work. There is no one right balance but discussion about the appropriate balance and the capacity to do something to change it, is evident. Fundholding has been a catalyst. Devolved budget responsibility does indeed seem to release innovation.

In a number of respects the flexibility is still not great enough. There are constraints on the kind of contracts GPs can make with community services. In 1993 the DoH effectively put a stop to fundholders contracting services to themselves through the agency of a private company. While some GPs may have abused this approach it had only grown up in the first place because the fundholding rules had prevented practices from paying themselves to do minor operations and treatments from the fund. There do certainly have to be safeguards and close monitoring of standards and outcomes, but done properly it can be more convenient for patients and usually much quicker.

In short, bottom-up budget flexibility has worked and should be given the chance to work better.

## Practice efficiency

One of the by-products of the additional managerial input needed to run the fund was, as we saw in Chapter 8, improved practice efficiency. The rest of the practices' activities come to be better managed too.

## Economy on drugs

Part of the scheme that is often overlooked is the inclusion of an element that covers the cost of drugs prescribed by the GP. If the practice saves money on this budget it can be used in the rest of the fund. This gives a direct incentive to GPs to review their prescribing habits carefully in a way that Government and commentators have been urging. The evidence from our regular interviews, discussed in Chapter 7, was that our sample GPs did devote serious attention to containing their drugs budgets. They did so more than non-fundholders, who did not face such direct incentives. We did not possess randomized control data to compare our practices' resulting drug spending with non-fundholders. However, we reviewed several studies that do suggest that fundholding GPs have not reduced the costs of their prescribing, but have increased the costs of their prescribing *more slowly* than non-fundholders. They seem to have done this by using more generic equivalents and being more cautious about taking up expensive new treatments.

## Administrative costs

The costs of practice-based contracting are clearly higher than the district-based contracting. The additional costs are to some extent offset by the clinical advantages that flow from the improved individualized patient information and monitoring of hospital progress that can be undertaken by the practice as a result. GP-based contracting seems to be better but to cost more.

## The scale of referrals

One original intention behind the thinking about GP fundholding was to make practices think more about the reasons for referring patients to hospital by facing the GP with the costs of each referral. If every GP were given similar budgets it might in the end reduce the wide and unexplained variability in GPs' referral patterns. In fact, the way the GPs' budgets have been set has not helped to achieve this goal. Because, as we describe in Chapter 8, budgets have been set on the basis of GPs' existing referral patterns, GPs have had no reason to revise their habits in this respect. The efficiency case for moving to a capitation-based fund allocation for this reason, as well as others, is strong, as we argue in Chapters 9 and 10.

### Perverse incentives for Trusts

We saw in Chapter 9 that setting GPs' budgets in a way that reflected local provider prices merely gave trusts the incentive to drive up the prices they charged fundholders. This reduced districts' budgets and perverted trusts' incentive structures. We have argued for tough regional cost conventions in fixing a formula-based budget for fundholders.

So far our conclusions have been largely favourable to this experiment in bottom-up GP-based purchasing. There is another side to the balance sheet.

### Comprehensive planning

Even if there are micro-efficiency gains to be reaped from having competitive purchasers, critics argue, the result is that districts lose their capacity to plan services for their populations. That requires one purchaser for the whole area. GP fundholders have fragmented any capacity to do this. They respond to patients' demands not the population's needs (Ham, 1992). They are less concerned with meeting the goals of *The Health of the Nation*. There is a series of answers to these claims, and some truth in them.

First, we have to remind ourselves yet again that, even with the inclusion of community services and 100 per cent coverage, fundholders potentially control no more than one-fifth of the combined hospital and community services' budget. In practice they have, in the past two years, controlled only 2 per cent, and now about 7 per cent, of that budget, and control over the community services element has been minimal. In most areas the argument is about fears not events.

Second, the concept of planning that districts tend to use in this argument is rooted in epidemiology and the past. The task of a district planner is seen to be examining trends in disease and populations at risk. Consumer preferences and patient demand are rude words or, at least, alien concepts. If they are to be used at all they involve patient questionnaires.

Private service organizations, however, have a quite different notion of planning. So, increasingly, do the new 'enabling' and contracting Social Service Departments. An organization like the supermarket chain Sainsburys uses trends in consumer preferences to tell them what consumers want. They also try to create demand and advertise heavily, but then so do health promotion agencies! As we saw in several of our examples, the more advanced districts were using the market choices of their GPs as valuable hard information in planning future services. The more obscurantist view is akin to the head office of Sainsbury responding to a changing pattern of sales by saying, 'It's those bloody customers again. They will keep changing their minds.'

This is not to say that epidemiology is not a valuable tool! But health experts' notions of 'need' pursued to the exclusion of consumer demand will kill the NHS. Take physiotherapy as an example. Most of our practices had used their fund to employ a physiotherapist for some sessions a week as a response to growing patient demand and minimal supply by community services or hospitals, except for patients recovering from an operation. Why was this service so neglected? The medical evidence shows it does no good, we were told. That was not the patients' view. It was the kind of response that drives people into the private sector. Without a balance of medical need *and* patient demand the service will not survive.

There is, nevertheless, substance in the argument. A clear priority has to be decided between the size of elective and emergency work. The GPs' budgets have been based, essentially, on what hospitals had been able to do three years ago rolled forward. Under much harsher budget pressure and growing emergency work a district might have to cut back its non-emergency cases for its non-fundholding patients. Fundholders' budgets for this kind of treatment were effectively ring fenced because they had been set on historic activity rates. This left a disparity between fundholding and non-fundholding patients' access to non-emergency care. The district could not deliver its priorities throughout its area.

In fact, by accident, fundholding may have been one way of

preserving budgets for treatments that relieve pain and disability rather than extend life at high cost. They may have produced a more rational allocation in some people's order of priority. Let us, however, assume that a district is right in its chosen balance between elective and non-elective surgery. The reason that there can be a clash is that the implied budgets for non-fundholding and fundholding GPs were set in different ways. If budgets for both sets of GPs were set on a common formula basis they would reflect whatever priority the district, in consultation with GPs, thought should be given to elective surgery. Within that broad heading the choice of *which* operations were given top priority could legitimately vary from one doctor to another, acting on their knowledge of patients' circumstances.

It must be said that relations between GP fundholders and districts in many areas *are* poor, and this does not make for good long-term planning. Districts and fundholders are realizing this and joint meetings and planning groups are emerging, especially where fundholding has developed most. We discuss this way forward below.

In contrast, we found that fundholding practices were more aware than they used to be of NHS-wide issues. They were more aware of financial issues and participated more in discussions about local priorities. This somewhat unexpected finding is consistent with Howie's (1993) findings in Scotland.

**Health of the Nation**

Given formula funding, the argument that fundholding interferes with reaching *Health of the Nation* targets falls away. It is in any case a weak point. It depends on the view that this is a district function. Yet all the 'key areas' mentioned in that document – coronary heart disease and stroke, cancer, mental illness, HIV/AIDS, accidents and the needs of the elderly, poor and black populations – have to rely on the GP as the critical link with the public. The more successful the GP fundholder is in reducing the illness of his or her patients, *given formula funding*, the more money the GP has to go round. This was always one of the main arguments for HMOs, on which fundholding was based. Non-fundholders gain less financial advantage from keeping their patients well. So, far from fundholding being at odds with *Health of the Nation*, it is a necessary adjunct to it. Since 1993, aiming at *Health of the Nation* goals has been a formal part of a fundholder's brief. It will be expected to figure in drawing up business plans, which have to be approved each year. Activities will include advice and screening sessions, which most of our practices did anyway. These strategies will need to be linked to FHSA and district priorities (Audit Commission, 1993a,b).

### Incentives for budget control

Early in 1993 (well before the end of the financial year), and again in August 1993 (early in the new financial year), hospitals in some areas began to run out of money to treat elective surgery patients paid for by districts. Fundholders' patients in these areas continued to be accepted. This was taken as evidence of unfairness in the money allocated to the fundholders. For the most part this was not the explanation. Hospitals had an incentive to get through as much work for their district as their capacity permitted them to do as fast as they could. When they finished their contracted total of procedures they would then hope to persuade the district to give them some more money to continue to treat patients. Publicity could only help bounce the district into giving more money. The politics of budgeting encouraged this kind of behaviour, just as it had under the old system. This time, however, the districts had some scapegoats.

In contrast, fundholders knew that if they ran out of funds early and had to turn patients away they might put patients off coming to a practice that could not order its own affairs. So, as we saw in Chapter 8, the practices husbanded their budgets rather well.

Our interviews with finance directors of district and trust hospitals showed that many would be happier with a system in which money actually did come with the patient. They would know where they were. As one finance director explained:

> It is all very well for districts to tell us we can only treat so many patients of this or that kind. Districts do not send us patients. GPs do. They drive our business. Districts do not. They are trying to second-guess demand and impose their own arbitrary limits . . . the sooner the people who take the decision to refer patients also have the cash to back their decision, the better it will be for us.

## Accountability

We have seen that large sums of public money, potentially much larger than now, will pass through the hands of private partnerships, which is the legal form GPs' 'firms' take. The fundholding budgets are formally ring fenced and held by FHSAs but there are ways in which 'leakage' can occur. One much publicized example is the private company. Another is the use of savings from the fund to extend the practice premises. This adds to the capital value of the practice, which partners buy into and sell when they move. Ingenious GPs will no doubt find other ways of leaking funds if a careful watch is not kept. In our experience, GPs had entered fundholding, with very few exceptions, because they cared about the quality of the service they could offer and were not driven by financial gain. However, accountability rules are for the exceptions and it is important they are tightened and properly implemented as the scheme grows. This point has been picked up by the Audit Commission (1993b).

## Budget volatility

One of the fears expressed before the scheme began (Weiner and Ferriss, 1990) was that practices would not be able to keep within their budgets. Emergencies and the random chance of having to meet a lot of high-cost patients in one year would drive them into the red, as had happened to American HMOs, they suggested. We have shown that this did not happen in the first two years. Practices may face more difficulty as cash limits tighten, but they possess the means to control their spending. The £5000 limit on practices' liabilities and the non-emergency nature of the categories covered had put fundholding on a much more secure footing than American HMOs.

Some have suggested that the scope of the fund should be extended to cover all hospital care. There are pilots taking place to test this (*Fundholding*, May 7 1993). They should be extended. The idea has virtues. It would extend the benefits of bottom-up funding to the whole range of hospital activity. It prevents fundholders shifting their patients into categories like emergency care not covered by the fund and it gives the GPs more power. However, the American evidence on budget volatility makes us very cautious about extending the fund outside controllable non-emergency care.

**In brief**

Our view is that what we have called bottom-up practice-based funding, for the areas of health care now covered by the fund, has provided tangible efficiency gains by the pressure it has exerted on hospitals and the innovation it has stimulated in practices themselves. Here we find ourselves in agreement with the Audit Commission (1993b). These gains are counterbalanced by the set of perverse incentives provided by the way the GPs' budgets are set. There is a perfectly feasible answer to this difficulty – the use of a formula-based budget allocation.

## THE EQUITY CRITERION

It is here that the major controversy surrounding fundholding has taken place. The main objection has been that fundholding has created a two-tier service. This is a confused claim that is based on a number of quite distinct propositions. Again some are valid and others not.

### More resources

At the heart of this case is the belief that the cash allocated to fundholding practices is greater than that available to similar non-fundholders for the 'purchase' of hospital and other services. The national and some regional comparisons we have seen do not bear this out. They suggest either that in the first two years there was little difference in the resources allocated on a national or regional basis and that some fundholders have probably been given less than a national or regional average allocation would have suggested. The application of the national average costs per capita for fundholding procedures suggested practices were getting approximately 15 per cent less than would have been expected. A more detailed study in Oxford Region showed a 9 per cent under-allocation, as we saw in Chapter 10.

On the other hand an analysis of districts in one county suggested fundholding practices had done rather better than they should; hospital service allocations were running at £76 per head in 1992–3 compared to a national average of £62. The hospital activity rates achieved by fundholders in the first wave had been 39.8 per 1000. This might well have been explained by their better contracting with more efficient hospitals. But the second-wavers achieved an activity rate of 51.7 per 1000, which was difficult to explain.

The fault seemed to lie in the way the base-line activity levels had been calculated on the basis of activity data sent in by the practices that was not checked back in detail with the providers. Fundholders had been counting some procedures as elective when the providers were counting them as emergency. They had counted in as fund-holding activity some procedures that were not properly in the list. Multiple procedures were sometimes counted as a single procedure by the hospital. The balance between day cases and inpatient and outpatient care was shifting in ways that the historic cost basis of funding would not reflect. Fourth-wave practice data would be subject to rigorous crosschecking with the providers' data. This had not been possible in the early years because of the poor hospital records.

One of our regions developed its own formula, finding a relationship between deprivation and unemployment and high demand for fundholding services. The national study did not find this. Nor was it clear that there was any very good medical reason to explain why unemployment should be linked to the range of procedures covered by fundholding. Fundholders in one county were getting more than the regional average on this basis but fundholders in two other areas were getting less. What seemed to be happening was that GPs in one area were well endowed with hospitals. They were getting more hospital services than patients in other areas. This held regardless of whether they were fundholders or not. All in all, it is difficult to support the contention that nationally GP fundholders were systematically overfunded compared to what a national formula would have given in the early years of the scheme. The impact of some local differential pricing with trusts charging fundholders higher prices may have been changing this conclusion in 1993–4.

As we saw in Chapter 9, the way in which budget setting has been undertaken has had perverse equity effects in some areas simply because the methods of budget setting for fundholders and non-fundholders have been different. In some areas they gained and in others they lost.

There can be no doubt that the case for formula funding is powerful on equity grounds as well as in terms of efficiency. It is certainly true that the size of the budgets allocated to different practices of the same size varied considerably. On a per patient basis we found some practices receiving half as much again as another practice. Yet these variations did no more than put £ signs on unequal uses of resources that were already taking place under the old system. By revealing them in economic terms they are made more difficult to sustain. The introduction of formula funding for access to non-emergency care, which is what GP fundholding essentially will do, will be a major step towards greater equity. At least, it will be if the same basis for allocation can be applied to non-fundholding practices.

## More management allowances and computing

Because practices are doing part of the contracting function and the administration of the funds requires more management and computing, fundholders have been given extra allowances to cover both kinds of costs. In a finite NHS budget this has to come from somewhere and non-fundholders understandably feel aggrieved, especially as these resources also spill over into all aspects of the practices' work. They argue that non-fundholding practices who wish to collaborate in locality purchasing schemes (see below) should have equivalent help.

## Queue jumping

This was the most inflammatory and complicated claim of all. On a simple level the belief was that consultants would pick fundholding patients from their waiting list and give them preference over non-fundholding patients. This was always implausible as a general strategy because it meant a hospital discriminating against the district, with whom it had a much larger contract. In a competitive system of annual contracts, any district with any sense would have stopped their contract with such a hospital.

In the first weeks of the new scheme it was claimed that one hospital was recommending such a policy to its staff. This immediately became a national 'scandal' and resulted in a joint agreement between the Royal Colleges and the DoH to the effect that consultants would be obliged to treat patients according to criteria of need and not which practice they came from. In some places informal arrangements seemed to be emerging where one consultant was prepared to deal with fundholders' contracts and others were not. This was a worrying development, but it reflected consultant reluctance to deal with fundholders.

GPs have always tried to make the best case they could for their patients, using past student days or whatever else might work. Most consultants' records could not distinguish who was a fundholding patient and who not, and it was far from clear that where they *did* know consultants were inclined to give preference to fundholding patients. We encountered several cases where consultants were hostile to patients when they found they were from a fundholding practice. In one case in the first year we found that local consultants had inexplicably found no high needs cases amongst fundholding patients after nine months while non-fundholders were being treated normally. The realization that this would lead to a complete withdrawal of contracts by fundholders produced a change. Markets actually resist such arbitrary treatment. It is administrative rationing that tends to do the reverse.

What the practices did do was to shop around, looking for hospitals, often some distance away, that could give a quicker service. This, of course, tends to even out the queues, taking patients from long waiting lists and adding them to shorter or faster-moving queues. Elementary economics tells us that the capacity to move and the knowledge of the market will tend to equalize queues and then to reduce them.

### Better purchasers, better services

Thus far we are unconvinced by the two-tier case. However, we have suggested, especially in Chapter 6, that fundholders have proved better purchasers than districts in some respects. Practice-based decisions, given the motivation and information base at that level, are simply better. If that is the case patients of fundholders will get gradually improved services. Some of that advantage will spin off onto non-fundholding practices, but not all. Small, non-fundholding practices unable to make the hospitals listen to them, will become even more disadvantaged than they are now. If fundholding is a better way of doing things and not all practices can become fundholders, there will increasingly become a gap between the two kinds of patient. Practices in poor areas with little energy or space to become fundholders were very poorly represented in the first waves.

To argue for the abolition of fundholding on this ground is, however, perverse. It is akin to the philosophical paradox that equality in human needs can best be achieved by starving everyone

(Goodin, 1990). Equity is best pursued by seeking to maximize opportunities, not to minimize them – levelling up not down (Le Grand, 1991). The conclusion to this logic is that a way has to be found of extending to non-fundholders the benefits of practice-based budgeting, as the Audit Commission (1993b, para 231) argued.

### Private sector

We have seen that one of the strongest motives for some to join fundholding has been to break free of local consultants whom GPs accused of not straining every nerve to reduce their long waiting lists in order to keep up the demand for their private clinics. In so far as this is true and fundholders break this tendency they will have had an impact on helping to break the really important two-tier system.

### Cream skimming

We discussed this at length in Chapter 11. Some patients have always been more trouble to GPs than others. Some are a very considerable trouble – the homeless are one such category – and GPs do not go out of their way to be welcoming to patients who may upset other patients or be a drain on the partners' time. Thus, to some extent cream skimming is not a new phenomenon. Fears that fundholding would sharply increase this tendency were based on the American literature we have discussed. In fact, because fundholders have been funded on a historic cost basis and really expensive patients' costs have been excluded, these fears have not been substantiated to any noticeable extent. At any rate, there is no hard evidence of cream skimming. Nevertheless, we established in Chapter 11 that it could become a reality as the Government moves to calculate GPs' budgets on a formula basis. Unless the formula includes factors that compensate for high-cost groups of patients, cream skimming may follow. We argued that it was possible and feasible to produce such a formula including the factors we isolated in Chapter 11. If we fail to counteract this incentive we shall have introduced a fatal virus into the NHS.

### In brief

There are justifiable fears that, left to grow as it is, and funded in a crude fashion, fundholding could offset its efficiency achievements with equity losses. This is not an inevitable outcome. There are measures that can be taken to spread the benefits of fundholding to all practices and to fund practices in an equitable way that will counteract any likely cream skimming tendencies.

## THE WAY FORWARD

There are ways to make fundholding more efficient and equitable.

### Formula funding

We argued that a new formula should include risk factors for patients in certain costly categories, e.g. diabetics. Practices could return information from their patient records giving details of the number of such patients and receive a higher allocation for them. This would have to be checked on a sample basis, and even so there are some dangers, but they do seem less dangerous than doing nothing.

### Extending the scheme and providing complementary alternatives

Some small practices may well be able to link up with larger fundholding practices and use their contracting expertise. Others may join a consortium. Many practices are, however, hostile to the whole idea of fundholding. In a number of areas GPs have come together to negotiate with hospitals as a group, with the help of their districts and FHSAs, not merely for fundholding procedures but more widely. This approach has come to be called 'locality purchasing' (Ham, 1993c). Districts were originally designed to be the agencies that were responsible for the management of their district general hospital and associated services. Now hospitals are separately managed, districts lose their logic. Contracting skills are scarce and are dissipated in numerous small purchasing areas. There has been an increasing tendency to amalgamate districts and this will go further with the slimming of administrative costs being pressed by the Government. In an attempt to keep a local input to contracting and to respond to the challenge set by GP fundholding some of the new larger groupings of district purchasers have introduced a lower local tier. This has taken different forms. In some places this merely amounts to 'outposted' district staff being responsible for a small area's needs and local consultation. In others, it amounts to groups of practices coming together to inform the purchasing agency of their purchasing needs. In a few areas practices may be given a shadow budget, rather like a fundholder's but covering most hospital services. The difference is that the GPs do not do the actual purchasing or have to keep within a clear budget limit. These schemes do reflect some aspects of GP fundholding but do not give autonomy or clear financial sanctions and incentives of the kind fundholding does.

An early informal example in one of our regions became a formal arrangement. A GP Forum advised the health authority on its purchasing strategy. Under a full formal scheme, a GP Commissioning Executive is now charged with identifying ways in which the district's broad contracts could be developed to meet special local needs identified by local GPs. These might be the need for more low-dependency beds in the local hospital, a diabetic day-care centre and more family-planning facilities. It would then be for the purchasing agency to implement the ideas in its contracts. The administrative costs of this devolved system of consultation could be met up to the level that would be given to a group of fundholders of the same size.

Many of the FHSAs are keen to develop a purchasing role on behalf of GPs who do not want to become fundholders, as well as advising those that do. One of our regions favoured boosting non-fundholders' influence on purchasing in this way as a means of evening up the influence of non-fundholders in the system.

A different approach to the same end had emerged in the county in our study with one of the highest percentages of fundholders. It was aimed at not only involving fundholders and non-fundholders in purchasing but also reaching an equitable allocation of finance between the two.

The county contained three district health authorities and one FHSA. It was decided to create a single commissioning agency joining the capacities of the three districts and the FHSA and linking up with GP fundholders to act as a single agency. This would not subsume or take over the functions of the fundholders but ensure that their preferences were included in the agency's planning. It had no statutory basis but the authorities agreed to delegate their powers to the agency. In this respect it was not unlike the Dorset Health Commission, created in 1992, and others. However, at its heart was the principle that each of the contracting parties should have equal resources available for the same purposes.

The aim is to develop a capitation formula for GP fundholders based on their population weighted for age and sex, as in the DoH's model, but adding morbidity and social deprivation factors. Exactly the same data would be collected for non-fundholding practices. They would then be allocated a shadow budget equal in size to what they would have received if they had been fundholders. Non-fundholders would then have a collective say in the scale and kind of contracts negotiated by the agency for non-fundholders in each of their localities. The next step would be to delegate to localities a shadow budget for the whole of the acute hospital budget. GPs would then be involved in discussing how much of the budget should go on non-emergency work covered by the fundholding scheme and how much to emergency work. Both sets of GPs would get the same split between emergency and fundholding procedures. Fundholders would negotiate on a practice basis for fundholding treatments and non-fundholders would negotiate collectively via the agency. Emergency care contracts would be negotiated collectively for all GPs in a locality. The intention was to bring the equal budgets into effect for 1994–5, devolving nominal activity budgets to non-fundholders by the end of 1993–4.

Our doubts about locality purchasing and budget holding are that localities do not in any real sense exist. GPs in an area have no shared legal responsibility or accountability. Their livelihood is not bound up in the viability of 'the locality'. They do not have the same shared responsibility to keep within the set budget. It was precisely these weaknesses that led to the collapse of loose American models of an equivalent kind that tried to act as HMOs without the shared legal responsibility for the budget. The great strength of GP fund-holding is that it is building on a well understood legal and social unit – the partnership.

## Competitive systems

The above plan seems to us to be based on the right kinds of principles, or at least the ones we have been advocating in this book, namely equal treatment and freedom for GPs to choose the kind of contracting regime that suits them best. This will bring alternative systems of contracting and groupings into competition. Patients could then choose which kind of purchaser they wished to act on their behalf.

The existence of fundholding has forced districts to come up with alternative systems of contracting. They may hope that it will make fundholding redundant. We doubt it. Many practices will want to preserve their independence. Some will prefer the new agency to do the contracting for them with consultation. Some GPs, of a collectivist frame of mind, will never have any truck with fundholding. So be it. Systems in competition will be good for patients.

# APPENDIX: THE SCOPE OF THE SCHEME

Below is the list of goods and services covered by the GP Fundholding scheme, as set out in Regulation 17(2) March 1993:

The Secretary of State for Health, in exercise of powers conferred by Regulation 17 (2) of the National Health Service (Fund-holding practices) (General) Regulations 1991 (SI 1991/ 582), hereby approves the goods and services, other than general medical services, specified in this list as being the goods and services which members of a recognised fund-holding practice may purchase for the individuals on the lists of patients of the members of the practice out of the allotted sum.

*1 Definitions*
(1) An 'in-patient' means a patient who has been admitted to hospital, whether or not he spends a night in the hospital.
(2) An 'out-patient' means a patient attending a hospital or clinic other than as an in-patient, or for whom a consultation by a hospital consultant is arranged by the GP in the patient's own home.
(3) An 'emergency' means where the patient is admitted to hospital when admission is unpredictable and at short notice.
(4) A 'GP' means a doctor who is providing general medical services under Part 11 of the National Health Service Act 1977.

*2*
(1) Subject to sub-paragraph (4), all goods and services listed in paragraph 3 provided to in-patients except in all cases

where the initial route of admission was an emergency or the patient had self-referred.

(2) For the goods and services listed in paragraph 3 the codes after each procedure are those found in the Office of Population Censuses and Surveys Tabular List of the Classifications of Surgical Operations and Procedures (Fourth Revision) published in February 1990.

(3) The allotted sum may not be applied to the provision of any of the goods and services listed in paragraph 3 for a patient who has been admitted to hospital before the date on which his GP becomes a member of a fund-holding practice.

*3 The goods and services referred to in paragraph 2(1) are:*
*Ophthalmology*
Operations for squint C31–35
Chalazion operation C12
Pterygium operation C39.1
* Extirpation of lesion of conjunctiva C39.2, C39.3, C39.4, C39.8, C39.9
Operations for ectropion, entropion, and ptosis C15.1, C15.2, C18
Operations for glaucoma C59, C60, C61, C62, C66.3, C66.4
* Extirpation of ciliary body C66.1, C66.2, C66.5, C66.8, C66.9
Operations for obstruction of the nasolacrimal duct C25, C27
Extraction of cataract with or without intra-ocular implant C71, C72, C74, C75
* Incision of capsule lens C73.1, C73.2, C73.3, C73.4, C73.8, C73.9
Corneal graft C46
Laser treatment for vascular retinopathies C82.1

*ENT*
Myringotomy D15.3
Insertion of grommet D15
Mastoidectomies D10 except D10.5
* Exenteration of mastoid air cells D10.5
Stapedectomy D17.1, D17.2
Tympanoplasty D14
Labyrinthectomy D26.2, D26.3
Septoplasty EO3.4–EO3.6

Sub-mucous resection of septum EO3.1
* Operations on septum of nose EO3.2, EO3.3, EO3.8, EO3.9
Polypectomy EO8.1
Ethmoidectomies E14.1–E14.4
Turbinectomy EO4.2–EO4.1
* Operations on turbinate of nose EO4.3, EO4.4, EO4.6, EO4.8, EO4.9
Cautery of lesion of nasal mucosa EO5.1
Puncture of maxillary antrum with wash-out E13.6
Drainage of maxillary sinus E12.2–E13.1
Exploration of frontal sinus E14.8
Tonsillectomy F34
Adenoidectomy E20.1
Pharyngoscopy E24, E25
Laryngoscopy E34, E35, E36
Laryngectomy E29
Block dissection T85.1

*Thoracic*
Bronchoscopy with or without biopsy E50, E51, E49, E48
Biopsy/excision of lesions of lung or bronchus E46.2–E46.9, E47.1, E55, E59.1–E59.3
Lobectomy E54
Pneumonectomy E54

*The cardiovascular system*
Operations for valvular or ischaemic disease of the heart K25–K35, K40–K51
(Excluding neonatal and infant surgery)

*General Surgery*
Partial thyroidectomy B12.1, B12.2, BO8.2–BO8.9
Total thyroidectomy BO8.1
* Other operations on thyroid gland B12.3, B12.4, B12.8, B12.9
Operation on salivary gland and ducts F44–F58
Operations on parathyroid glands B14, B16
Oesophagoscopy with or without endoscopic procedures G14–G19
Dilation of oesophagus G15.2, G15.3, G18.2, G18.3
Operations on varices of the oesophagus G10, G14.4, G17.4

Gastrectomy partial or total G27, G28

Vagotomy with or without other operative procedures A27±G33.1, G40.1, G40.3

Endoscopy with or without endoscopic procedures G43–G45, G54–G55, G62, G64, G65, G79, G80

Laparoscopy with or without biopsy T42, T43

Excision of lesion of small intestine G50, G53.1, G59, G63.1, G70, G78.1

Partial colectomy H06–H11

Total colectomy H04, H05

Sigmoidectomy with or without biopsy/polypectomy H23–H28

Colonoscopy with or without biopsy/polypectomy H20–H22

Exteriorisation of bowel H14, H15

Repair of prolapsed bowel H35, H36, H42

Operations for anal fissure and fistula H55, H56.4

Excision of rectum H33

Pilonidal sinus H59, H60

Dilation of anal sphincter H54

Haemorrhoidectomy H51–H53

Operations of the gall bladder J18–J26

Laparoscopic cholecystectomy J18.3, Y50.8

Operations on the bile ducts J27–J52

Mastectomy B27

Excision/biopsy of breast lesion B28, B32

Operations on duct of breast B34

Repair of inguinal hernia T19–T21

Repair of femoral hernia T22, T23

Repair of incisional hernia T25, T26

Varicose veins stripping/ligation (including injections) L85–L87

Surgical treatment of ingrowing toenail S64, S68, S70.1

Excision/biopsy of skin or subcutaneous tissues S05, S06, S09, S10.2, S11.2, S13–S15

\* Curettage of lesion of skin S08.1, S08.2, S08.3, S08.8, S08.9

\* Other destruction of lesion of skin of head or neck S01.1, S01.3, S01.4, S01.8, S01.9

\* Other destruction of lesion of skin on other site S11.1, S11.3, S11.4, S11.8, S11.9

Lymph node excision biopsy T87

*Genito-urinary*
Cystoscopy with or without destruction of lesion bladder M42, M44, M45, M76, M77
Dilatation of urethra/urethrotomy M58, M76.4, M81, M79, M76.3, M75.3
Urethroplasty M73
Open repair M73.4
Prostatectomy open or TUR M61, M65
Operation on hydrocele N11
Orchidopexy N08, N09
Male sterilisation N17
Circumcision N30
Varicocele N19
Removal of ureteric or renal calculus M26–M28, M09, M06.1, M23.1
Lithotripsy M14, M31
Nephrectomy M02, M03

*Gynaecology*
Oophorectomy/salpingoophorectomy Q22.1, Q22.3, Q23.1, Q23.2, Q23.5, Q23.6, Q24.1, Q24.3
* Unilateral excision of adnexa of uterus Q23.3, Q23.4, Q23.8, Q23.9
Ovarian cystectomy Q43.2
Wedge resection of ovary Q43.1
* Partial excision of ovary Q43.3, Q43.8, Q43.9
Diagnostic laparoscopy with or without biopsy Q39, Q50
Female sterilisation Q27, Q28, Q35, Q36
Patency tests of fallopian tubes Q41, Q39.9
Hysterectomy abdominal/vaginal Q07, Q08
Myomectomy Q09.2
D and C with or without polypectomy Q10.3
EUA Q55.2
Hysterectomy/endometrial resection Q17, Q18
Cone biopsy Q03.1–Q03.3
Colposcopy with or without biopsy of cervix P27.3, Q02, Q03.4, Q03.9
* Biopsy of cervix uteri Q03.5, Q03.8, Q03.9
Anterior or posterior repair (including vault prolapse, amputation of cervix, perineorrhaphy, colpsuspension) P22, P23, P24, P13.2, P13.3

Vulvectomy/partial vulvectomy/vulval biopsy P05, P06, P09.1
Marsupialisation of Bartholin's cyst/abscess P03.2, P05.3

*Orthopaedics*
Operation on intervertebral discs V29–V35, V52
Therapeutic lumbar epidural injection A52.1
Arthroplasty/revision arthroplasty of hip or knee W37–W42,
W46–W48
Upper tibial osteotomy W12+, Z77.4
Arthroplasty with or without other intra-articular procedures
W82–W88
Intra-articular injections aspiration W90
Menisectomy W82, W70
Osteotomy for hallus valgus/rigidus W57.1, W15
Correction of hammer toe W59.5
* Fusion of interphalangeal joint of great toe W59.4
Dupuytren's contracture T52.1, T52.2
Carpal tunnel decompression A65.1
Release of trigger finger (tenovaginitis) T72.3
Excision of ganglion T59, T60
* Operations on bursa T62.6, T62.8, T62.9
Aspiration/excision of bursa T62.1–T62.5
Removal of internal fixation from bone W28.3
Soft tissue operations on joint toe W79

*4*
(1) Subject to sub-paragraph (2), all goods and services pro-
    vided to out-patients where:
    (a) these goods and services are listed in paragraph 5
        and
    (b) a tick appears against those goods and services in
        column A of paragraph 5.
(2) Notwithstanding sub-paragraph (1), the goods and ser-
    vices listed in paragraph 5 are not goods and services which
    may be purchased for patients of members of fund-holding
    practices if:
    (a) a tick appears against those goods and services in
        Column B of paragraph 5, or
    (b) the goods and services were provided following any
        case where the initial route of admission was as an
        emergency or the patient had self-referred.

5   *The goods and services referred to in paragraph 4 are*

|  |  | Column A Applicable | Column B Not Applicable |
|---|---|---|---|
| a. | Out-patient treatment | | |
| | i) in general | + | |
| | ii) first out-patient appointment where treatment follows or is a direct result of a procedure listed in paragraph 3 | + | |
| | iii) first out-patient appointment where treatment follows or is a direct result of an in-patient stay not listed in paragraph 3 | | + |
| | iv) first appointment following an in-patient stay that commenced prior to the practice becoming a fund-holder. | | + |
| | v) all appointments thereafter | + | |
| | vi) chemotherapy and radiotherapy provided on a day case or out-patient basis | | + |
| | vii) renal dialysis | | + |
| | viii) all out-patient treatment at a Genito-Urinary Medicine Clinic. | | + |
| b. | Diagnostic tests and investigations provided on out-patient basis | | |
| | i) in general | + | |
| | ii) breast screening carried out under the national call and recall programme and consequential tests or investigations (The national call and recall programme whereby every woman aged between 50 and 64 is invited to attend for screening by mammography and is recalled for screening every 3 years) | | + |

|  | Column A Applicable | Column B Not Applicable |
|---|---|---|

iii) cervical screening carried out under the national call and recall prográmme (The national call and recall programme is a national programme whereby every woman aged between 20 and 64 is invited to attend for cervical screening and is recalled at least every 5 years) — Column B: +

iv) diagnostic follow-up of an abnormal smear from b. iii. — Column A: +

v) issue of hearing aids following an audiological test — Column B: +

vi) where any diagnostic test or investigation is carried out by the Public Health Laboratory. — Column B: +

c. Services to which a GP may refer directly, or where the referral has en ordered by a hospital consultant following referral by a GP

i) physiotherapy, speech therapy, occupational therapy, chiropody and dietetics — Column A: +

ii) services in c. i above where these are supplied by the Social Services Department of the Local Authority or by the Local Education Authority. — Column B: +

d. Maternity services

i) In general, including post-natal care — Column B: +

ii) pregnancy tests — Column A: +

iii) antenatal blood tests — Column A: +

iv) services under d. iii. above provided as part of an out-patient appointment. — Column B: +

|  |  | Column A Applicable | Column B Not Applicable |
|---|---|---|---|
| e. | Domiciliary consultations | | |
|  | i)  consultations by a hospital consultant arranged by the GP. | + | |
| f. | Community nursing services | | |
|  | i)  health visiting services for patients of the practice | + | |
|  | ii)  public health element of health visiting | | + |
|  | iii)  district nursing services for patients of the practice | + | |
|  | iv)  public health element of district nursing | | + |
|  | v)  referrals to health visitors/ district nurses from other agencies | + | |
|  | vi)  referrals for specialist nursing services. | | + |
| g. | Mental health services | | |
|  | i)  counselling | + | |
|  | ii)  referrals to all members of the mental health care team (whether as a member of the team or individually) including consultant psychiatrists, CPNs, psychotherapists, psychologists, but excluding psychiatric social worker | + | |
|  | iii)  referrals to mental health care team from other agencies | | + |
|  | iv)  NHS services for people with learning disabilities (PLD) | + | |
|  | v)  referrals for services for PLD from other agencies | + | |
|  | vi)  local authority services for PLD. | | + |

(* denotes amendments to the scope of the scheme which will be implemented 1 April 1994.)

A brief outline of the other main Department of Health publications and circulars that have been issued since the inception of the GP fundholding scheme are listed below in chronological order.

*Funding General Practice (booklet), December 1989*
This booklet gives a general introduction to the fundholding scheme to interested GPs and practices.

*Guidance on Contracting by Fundholders, February 1991*
This document explains how GP fundholders' contracts should be set in the first year of the scheme. As well as being aimed at fundholders, this document is intended to inform district health authorities, regional health authorities, family health service authorities and provider units about the contracting process.

*General Practice Funding: Financial Matters (EL(91)36), March 1991*
This document explains the responsibilities of regional health authorities and family health service authorities which relate to fundholding.

*Draft Guidance on Fundholders Purchasing and Selling Services, May 1991*
This document discusses concerns about limited companies which some fundholding practices have set up under the scheme. It has been superseded by *GP Fundholding Practices: The Provision of Secondary Care (HSG(93)14) March 1993* (see below).

*Joint Guidance for Consultants on GP Fundholding (EL(91)84), June 1991*
This document provides guidance for providers and consultants that aims to prevent the disadvantage of some patients over and above that of another purchasers' patients. It stresses that all patients should get the same standard of clinical care regardless of the form of contract that providers set with purchasing authorities, including GP fundholders. The principle of treatment according to clinical need is to be recognized within the contracting framework and, to achieve this, hospital consultants must have full involvement in the contracting process. It states that providers should have a common waiting list for seriously ill patients and for highly specialized diagnosis and treatment.

*Priorities and Planning Guidance 1993–4 (EL(92)47), July 1992*
This document sets out the key priorities of the NHS and gives

guidance on how purchasers and providers should achieve them. The key priorities are: (1) implementing *Health of the Nation*; (2) developing the Patient's Charter; and (3) together with local authorities, providing high quality social and health care in the community. It is emphasized that purchasers, including fund-holders, should collaborate and establish alliances with other agencies in the community so that objectives can be met. (See below, *Priorities and Planning Guidance 1994–5 (EL(93)54) June 1993*.)

*Guidance on the Extension of the Hospital and Community Health Services Elements of the Scheme from 1 April, 1993 (EL(92)48), July 1992* (the 'Yellow Book')
This guidance sets out in detail the rules governing the extension of the hospital and community health services element of the fund. It states that in setting budgets for community nursing, regions will need to consider as a baseline the current level of service provided to each practice, as well as the cost of providing these services. The guidance also sets out regulations that state strictly that practices are required to place contracts for community nursing with established NHS providers and are not able to directly employ nurses or use private providers. However, practices are not obliged to use community services providers that they have used in the past. In contract setting, practices are also limited to using fixed price non-attributable contracts for community nursing. (See below, *Supplementary Guidance (HSG(92)53) December 1992*.)

*GP Fundholders: Public Availability of Contracts (EL(92)68), October 1992*
This document states that one of the aims of the Patient's Charter is to improve the access to information for the public. Patients should be able to have access to contracts that fundholders have set with providers; these should be made available via district health authorities.

*General Practice Fundholding: Guidance on Setting Budgets for 1993–4 (EL(92)83), November 1992*
This guidance sets out the reason for moving from a purely historic basis for calculating budgets and explains how budgets will be set in the future with the introduction of capitation benchmarks into budget negotiations.

*Extension of the Hospital and Community Health Services Elements of the GP Fundholding Scheme – Supplementary Guidance (HSG(92)53), December 1992*
This circular offers further guidance on the extension of the GP fundholding scheme set out in document EL(92)48 (the 'Yellow book'). It clarifies the range of services to be included and in particular discusses in some detail, health services for patients with learning disabilities.

This supplementary guidance also sets out the responsibilities of fundholders under the Children Act 1989. It stresses that fundholders have a responsibility to co-operate and liaise with Social Services Departments to assist them in carrying out their duties under the Act.

Included in the annexe of this document are negotiating issues that fundholders may consider and specimen contracts that relate to the extension of the scheme. (See also, *Health Services for People with Learning Disabilities (mental handicap) (HSG(92)42) October 1992.*)

*Tertiary Referrals (EL(92)97), December 1992*
This document states that from 1 April 1993 providers in England will no longer be required to obtain prior authorization from the appropriate purchasing authority or GP fundholder before accepting for treatment tertiary referral patients who have not been referred within existing contracts. Instead, consultants initiating a tertiary extra-contractual referral will be required to inform the relevant purchasing authority or GP fundholder when the referral is made. Purchasers will be expected to meet the cost of treatment. (See below, *Guidance on Operation of Notification Arrangements for Extra-Contractual Referrals (HSG(93)8) February 1993.*)

*Manual of Accounts, version 2.0 (FDL(93)16), February 1993*
This document replaces version (1.0) of the manual of accounts and includes the extension of the scheme. The manual is aimed primarily at the practice manager or administrator and any professional adviser whose services may be employed by the practice. It explains the budgetary process and sets out how the fund should be operated.

*1992–93 End of Year Arrangements for All Purchasers (Including GP Fundholders) (FDL(93)08), February 1993*
All purchasers, including GP fundholders, are asked to work

together in order to reduce end-of-year adjustments and accruals caused by delayed payments and invoicing. It recognizes that problems in the information and invoicing flows between providers and GP fundholders have resulted in difficulties in agreeing accounts for 1991–2. The letter proposes a course of action as to how cash-flow problems could be reduced.

*Guidance on Operation of Notification Arrangements for Tertiary Extra-Contractual Referrals (HSG(93)8), February 1993*
This document gives further details about the changes set out in EL(92)97 (see above) which states that providers no longer require authorization before accepting tertiary extra-contractual referrals. This will only apply to tertiary extra-contractual referrals made from one NHS provider to another. Excluded are tertiary referrals to non-designated units for services designated under the supra-regional service arrangements. It is still necessary to obtain prior authorization from the purchasing authority for a non-emergency extra-contractual referral that is not a tertiary referral.

This document also sets out guidance for good practice and includes a specimen notification form.

*List of Goods and Services Covered by the GP Fundholding Scheme Reg. 17.2, March 1993*
This document defines the list of goods and services which the members of a fundholding practice may purchase out of their allotted fund. It consolidates changes announced in the 'Yellow Book' under cover of EL(92)48 and replaces the original list of goods and services (see above).

*GP Fundholding Practices: The Provision of Secondary Care (HSG(93)14), March 1993*
From 1 April 1993, the NHS (Fund-holding Practices) Regulations 1993 will allow GP fundholders to be paid from the fund for providing a specified range of non-general medical services to their own patients. These revised arrangements replace the system of setting up limited companies to provide services under contract to the fund. This guidance sets out the services to be covered and the criteria that regions should use in assessing proposals for providing these services from fundholders and their subsequent monitoring arrangements.

*The National Health Service (Fund-holding Practices) Regulations 1993, Statutory Instrument No.567, March 1993*
This contains the legal requirements governing GP fundholding with effect from 1 April 1993. It covers the procedure for the application for recognition as a fundholding practice and sets out the regulations as to how fundholding practices may use their allotted fund. Included in this document are the procedures for the removal of recognition of fundholding status and the rules relating to a practice wishing to leave the scheme.

*Priorities and Planning Guidance 1994–5 (EL(93)54), 29 June 1993*
This document sets out the policy framework for all purchasers, including GP fundholders, within which purchasing authorities manage the service. Strategies for improving health are a priority as well as providing better services and giving value for money. These aims should be reflected in purchasing plans and targets should be set and monitored against specified success criteria. It stresses the importance of effective purchasing and sets out initiatives to guide this process. In particular, the development of five-year purchasing strategies should be worked towards and all contracts must contain indicative volumes.

*GP Fundholding: management allowances (HSG(93)43), August 1993*
This document provides guidance on entitlement to and payment of the GP fundholding management allowances.

Eligible practices are able to claim a management allowance in their preparatory year, this amounts to £17,500, or £20,000 if two or more practices have grouped together to meet the list size criteria for managing a fund. Once a practice is granted fundholding status, they are able to claim up to a maximum of £35,000 management allowances in each fundholding year.

The guidance also sets out expenses covered by management allowances that regional health authorities will agree to reimburse.

# REFERENCES

Akerlof, G.A. (1970). 'The market for "lemons": qualitative uncertainty and the market mechanism', *Quarterly Journal of Economics*, *84*(3), 488–500.

Ash, A., Porell, F., Gruenberg, L., Sawitz, E. and Beiser, A. (1989). 'Adjusting Medicare capitation payments using prior hospitalization data', *Health Care Financing Review*, *10*(4), 17–29.

Audit Commission (1993a). *Practices Make Perfect: The Role of the Family Health Services Authority*. London, HMSO.

Audit Commission (1993b). *Their Health Your Business: The Role of the District Health Authority*. London, HMSO.

Barr, N., Glennerster, H. and Le Grand, J. (1988). *Reform and the NHS*, Welfare State Discussion Paper WSP/32. London, London School of Economics.

Bradlow, J. and Coulter, A. (1993). 'Effect of NHS reforms on general practitioners' referral patterns', *British Medical Journal*, *306*, 433–7.

Brown, L.D. (1983). *Politics and Health Care Organisation: HMOs as federal policy*. Washington DC, Brookings Institution.

Burr, A.J., Walker, R., and Stent, S.J. (1992). 'Impact of fundholding on general practice prescribing patterns', *Pharmaceutical Journal*, 24 October.

Butler, J. (1992). *Patients, Policies and Politics: before and after Working for Patients*. Buckingham: Open University Press.

Crump, B.J., Cubbon, J.E., Drummond, M.F., Hawkes, R.A. and March-ment, M.D. (1991). 'Fundholding in general practice and financial risk', *British Medical Journal*, *302*, 1582–4.

Culyer, A.J. and Posnett, J.W. (1990). 'Hospital behaviour and competition', in *Competition in Health Care: reforming the NHS*, Culyer, A.J., Maynard, A.K. and Posnett, J.W. (eds). London, Macmillan.

Day, P. (1992). 'The state, the NHS, and general practice', *Journal of Public Health Policy*, *13*(2).

Department of Health (1989a). *Working for Patients*. London, HMSO.

Department of Health (1989b). *Practice Budgets for General Medical Practitioners*. London, HMSO.

Department of Health (1990). *General Practice Fundholders' Manual of Accounts*. London, HMSO.

Department of Health (1991). *Patient's Charter*. London, HMSO.

Department of Health (1992). *The Health of the Nation*. London, HMSO.

Department of Health and Social Services (1987). *Promoting Better Health*. London, HMSO.

Duan, N., Manning, W.G., Morris, C.N. and Newhouse, J.P. (1983). 'A comparison of alternative models of the demand for medical care', *Journal of Business and Economic Statistics*, *1*(2), 115–26.

Dunleavy, P. (1991). *Democracy, Bureaucracy and Public Choice*. Hemel Hempstead, Harvester Wheatsheaf.

Dutch Government Committee on Choices in Health Care (1992). *Choices in Health Care*. Zoetermeer, the Netherlands, Ministry of Welfare, Health and Cultural Affairs.

Dutch Ministry of Welfare, Health and Cultural Affairs (1988). *Changing Health Care in the Netherlands*. Amsterdam, Dutch Ministry of Welfare.

Elmore, R.F. (1978). 'Organisational models of social program implementation', *Public Policy*, *26*, 185–228.

Elmore, R.F. (1982). 'Backward mapping: implementation research and policy decisions', in *Studying Implementation*, Williams, W. *et al.* (eds). Chatham, NJ, Chatham House.

Enthoven, A. (1985). *Reflections on the Management of the NHS*. London, Nuffield Trust.

Epstein, A.M. and Cumella, E.J. (1988). 'Capitation payment: using predictors of medical utilization to adjust rates', *Health Care Financing Review*, *10*(1), 51–69.

Glennerster, H. (1992). *Paying for Welfare: the 1990s*. Hemel Hempstead, Harvester Wheatsheaf.

Glennerster, H. and Matsaganis, M. (1992). *The English and Swedish Health Care Reforms*, Welfare State Discussion Paper WSP/79. London, London School of Economics.

Glennerster, H., Matsaganis, M. and Owens, P. (1992). *A Foothold for Fundholding*. London, King's Fund Institute.

Goodin, R.E. (1990). 'Relative needs' in *Needs and Welfare*, Goodin, R.E. and Ware, A. (eds). London, Sage.

Hall, P., Parker, R.A. and Webb, A. (1975). *Change, Choice and Conflict in Social Policy*. London, Heinemann.

Ham, C. (1992). *Learning from Experience: the next steps in implementing the NHS reforms*. Text of a speech given at the Institute of Health Service Managers Conference, 5 March 1992. Available from Health Services Management Centre, Birmingham University.

Ham, C. (1993a). 'How go the NHS reforms?', *British Medical Journal*, *306*, 77–8.

Ham, C. (1993b). 'Reviewing the NHS Review', *British Medical Journal*, *307*, 5–6.

Ham, C. (1993c). *Locality Purchasing*. Birmingham: Health Services Management Centre, University of Birmingham.

Higgins, J. (1993). 'Merger on the Orient Express', *Health Service Journal*, *26 August*.

Hill, M. (1993). *The Policy Process: a reader*. Hemel Hempstead, Harvester Wheatsheaf.

Hills, J. (1993). *The Future of Welfare: A guide to the debate*. York, Rowntree Foundation.

Hirschman, A.O. (1970). *Exit, Voice and Loyalty: responses to decline in firms, organisations and states*. Cambridge, MA, Harvard University Press.

Howie, J.G.R. (1992). 'The Scottish general practice shadow fund-holding project – outline of an evaluation', *Health Bulletin*, *50, 4 July*, 316–28.

Howie, J.G.R. (1993). 'Evaluation of the Scottish shadow fund-holding project: first results', *Health Bulletin*, *51*(2), 94–105.

Howland, J., Stokes, J., Crane, S.C. and Belanger, A.J. (1987). 'Adjusting capitation using chronic disease factors: a preliminary study', *Health Care Financing Review*, *9*(2), 15–23.

Hurst, J. (1991). 'Reforming health care in seven European nations', *Health Affairs*, *10*(3), 7–21.

Israeli State Commission of Enquiry into the Israeli Health Care System (1991). *Report*. Jerusalem, Ministry of Health.

Jowell, R., Witherspoon, S. and Brook, L. (1989). *British Social Attitudes: Special International Report*. Aldershot, Gower.

Keeley, D. (1993). 'The fundholding debate: should practices reconsider the decision not to fundhold?', *British Medical Journal*, *306*, 697–8.

Lambert, R. (1963). *Sir John Simon 1816–1904 and English Social Administration*. London, MacGibbon and Kee.

Le Grand, J. (1982) *The Strategy of Equality*. London, Allen and Unwin.

Le Grand, J. (1991). *Equity and Choice*. London, HarperCollins.

Le Grand, J. and Bartlett, W. (1993). *Quasi Markets and Social Policy*. London, Macmillan.

Le Grand, J., Glennerster,H. and Maynard, A. J. (1991) 'Quasi markets and social policy', *Economic Journal*, *Vl 101*(408), 1256–88.

Letwyn, O. and Redwood, J. (1988). *Britain's Biggest Enterprise*. London, Centre for Policy Studies.

Lipsky, M. (1980). *Street Level Bureaucracy: dilemmas of the individual in public services*. New York, Russell Sage Foundation.

Lubitz, J., Beebe, J. and Riley, G. (1985). 'Improving the Medicare HMO payment formula to deal with biased selection', in *Advances in Health Economics and Health Services Research 6*, 101–122, Scheffler, R. and Rossiter, L. (eds). Greenwich, CN, JAI Press.

Luft, H.S. (1986). 'Compensating for biased selection in health insurance', *Milbank Quarterly*, *64*(4), 566–91.

Luft, H. and Miller, R.H. (1988). 'Patient selection in a competitive health system', *Health Affairs*, 7(3), 97–119.

McAvoy, B. (1993). 'Heartsink hotel revisited', *British Medical Journal*, 306, 375–8.

Maddala, G.S. (1988). *Introduction to Econometrics*. New York, Macmillan.

Martin, J.P. (1957). *Social Aspects of Prescribing*. London, Heinemann.

Matsaganis, M. and Glennerster, H. (1993). 'Patient characteristics as determinants of hospital expenditure in general practice fund-holding', *Commissioning for Health Conference*, York, Health Economists Study Group and Faculty of Public Health Medicine.

Matsaganis, M. and Glennerster, H. (1994). 'The threat of "cream skimming" in the post-reform NHS'. *Journal of Health Economics 13*, 31–60.

Maxwell, M., Heaney, D., Howie, J.R.G. and Noble, S. (1993). 'General practice fundholding: observations on prescribing patterns and costs using the defined daily dose method', *British Medical Journal, 307*, 1190–94.

Maynard, A. (1986). 'Performance incentives in general practice', in *Health Education and General Practice*, Teeling Smith, G. (ed). London, Office of Health Economics.

Newhouse, J.P. (1982). 'Is competition the answer?', *Journal of Health Economics*, 1(1), 109–16.

Newhouse, J.P. (1986). 'Rate adjusters for Medicare under capitation', *Health Care Financing Review*, Annual Supplement, 45–55.

Newhouse, J.P., Manning, W.G., Keeler, E.B. and Sloss, E.M. (1989). 'Adjusting capitation rates using objective health measures and prior utilization', *Health Care Financing Review, 10*(3), 41–54.

Newton, J., Fraser, M., Robinson, J., and Wainwright, D. (1993). 'Fundholding in Northern Region: the first year', *British Medical Journal, 306*, 375–8.

OECD (1987). *Financing and Delivering Health Care*. Paris, Organisation for Economic Co-operation and Development.

OECD (1992a). *Market Type Mechanisms*, Occasional Papers in Public Management, No 1. Paris, Organisation for Economic Co-operation and Development.

OECD (1992b). *The Reform of Health Care*. Paris, Organisation for Economic Co-operation and Development.

Osborne, D. and Gaebler, T. (1992). *Reinventing Government: How the Entrepreneurial Spirit is Transforming the Public Sector from School-house, City Hall to the Pentagon*. Reading, MA, Addison Wesley.

Owens, P. and Glennerster, H. (1990). *Nursing in Conflict*. London, Macmillan.

Pirie, M. and Butler, E. (1988). *The Health of Nations*. London, Adam Smith Institute.

Power, A. (1987). *Property before People*. London, Allen and Unwin.

Propper, C. (1993). 'Quasi-Markets contracts and quality in health and social care: the US experience', in *Quasi Markets and Social Policy*, Le Grand, J. and Bartlett, W. (eds). London, Macmillan.

Reekie, W.D. and Weber, M.H. (1979). *Profits, Politics and Drugs*. London, Macmillan.

Robinson, J.C., Luft, H.S., Gardner, L.B. and Morrison, E.M. (1991). 'A method for risk-adjusting employer contributions to competing health insurance plans', *Inquiry*, *28*, 107–16.

Robinson, R. (1988). *Efficiency and the NHS: a case for an internal market?* London, Institute for Economic Affairs.

Robinson, R. and Le Grand, J. (eds) (1994). *Evaluating the National Health Service Reforms*. London, King's Fund.

Roland, M.O., Bartholemew, J., Morrell, D.C., McDermott, A. and Paul, E. (1990). 'Understanding hospital referral rates: a user's guide', *British Medical Journal*, *301*, 98–102.

Rothschild, M. and Stiglitz, J. (1976). 'Equilibrium in competitive insurance markets: an essay on the economics of imperfect information', *Quarterly Journal of Economics*, *90*(4), 629–49.

Sainsbury Committee (1967). *Report of the Committee into the relationship of the pharmaceutical industry with the National Health Service 1965–7*. London, HMSO.

Saltman, R.B. and von Otter, C. (1992). *Planned Markets and Public Competition: Strategic reform in northern European health systems*. Buckingham, Open University Press.

Scheffler, R. (1989). 'Adverse selection: the Achilles heel of the NHS reforms', *Lancet*, 29 April. 950–2.

Schultze, C.L. (1968). *The Politics and Economics of Public Spending*. Washington DC, Brookings Institution.

Swedish Committee on the Funding and Organisation of Health Services and Medical Care (1993). *Three Models for Health Care Reform in Sweden*, A Report from the Expert Group. Stockholm, Ministry of Health and Social Affairs.

Taylor-Gooby, P. and Lawson, R. (1993). *Markets and Managers: New Issues in the Delivery of Welfare*. Buckingham, Open University Press.

Thatcher, M. (1993). *The Downing Street Years*. London: HarperCollins.

van Vliet, R.C.J.A. and van de Ven, W.P.M.M. (1990). How can we prevent cream skimming in a competitive health insurance market? Zurich, Second World Congress on Health Economics.

Wallack, S.S., Tompkins, C.P. and Gruenberg, L. (1988), 'A plan for rewarding efficient HMOs', *Health Affairs*, *7*(3), 80–96.

Weiner, J. and Ferriss, P. (1990). *GP budget holding in the UK: lessons from America*, Research Report 7. London, King's Fund Institute.

Welch, W.P. (1985). 'Medicare capitation payments to HMOs in light of regression toward the mean in health care costs', *Advances in Health Economics and Health Services Research* (R. Scheffler and L. Rossiter), *6*, 75–96. Greenwich, CN, JAI Press.

White House Domestic Policy Council (1993). *The President's Health Security Plan*. New York, Times Books.

Willetts, D. and Goldsmith, M. (1988). *Managed Health Care: a new system for a better NHS*. London, Centre for Policy Studies.

# INDEX

**FINANCING HEALTH CARE IN THE 1990s**

**John Appleby**

The British National Health Service has embarked on a massive programme of change in the way it provides health care. The financing of the Health Service is at the heart of this change and controversies over this issue are likely to stay with us in the coming decade, whichever political party is in power. This book explores some of the directions that the financing of health care could take over the next ten years. For instance, will the Conservative Government's stated commitment to a health care system financed out of general taxation remain? Or, if the current reforms fail to bring measurable benefits of any significance, will the political pressures to take reforms even further lead to still greater changes in funding, financing and operations? Will the state of the national economy necessitate further reforms? Or might the reforms to date take an uncharted path, with some unexpected outcomes?

For the senior student, academic or health care professional this book offers an expert's view of the financing of the Health Service now and in the future.

*Contents*
*New directions – Seeds of change – Past trends in health-care funding – The right level of funding – A market for health care – Managing the market: the US experience – Managing the market: the West German experience – Some views of the future – Conclusions – References – Index.*

192 pp      0 335 09776 6 (Paperback)      0 335 09777 4 (Hardback)

**PATIENTS, POLICIES AND POLITICS**
BEFORE AND AFTER *WORKING FOR PATIENTS*

**John Butler**

The 1989 White Paper *Working for Patients* was the watershed of the Conservative Government's policymaking for the future of the British National Health Service. This book examines the political and historical background to the White Paper, its contents and proposals, and the actions and reactions to which it gave rise. The book is written in an accessible and jargon-free style and is aimed at a wide range of readers from various professional and academic backgrounds who are seeking a synoptic and balanced view of this remarkable episode in the history of the NHS.

***Contents***
*Origins – Context – Content – Purposes – Dissent – Prophecies – Implementation – Reflections – References – Index.*

160 pp     0 335 15647 9 (Paperback)     0 335 15648 7 (Hardback)

## PUBLIC LAW AND HEALTH SERVICE ACCOUNTABILITY
**Diane Longley**

This book examines the relationship between the processes of account-ability and management within the health service in the light of the recent National Health Service and Community Care Act. The author argues that health care is a social entitlement, to be moulded and allocated according to rational social choices and to be protected from becoming a commodity which is largely controlled by unaccountable market forces. Insufficient attention has been given to the potential role of law in the shaping of health policy and the management of the health service as a public organization. The arguments put forward here rest on a firm belief in a constitutional backcloth for the operation of all government and public services. The author calls for greater openness in health policy planning, in management and professional activities, the introduction of standards of conduct in health service management and for the establishment of an independent 'Institute of Health' to analyse and advise on health policy.

This important and timely book will be of interest to a wide range of students, academics and professionals interested in health service policy, politics and management.

*Contents*
*Diagnostic deficiencies: health policy, public law and public management –*
*Prescriptive dilemmas: accountability and the statutory and administrative*
*structure of the NHS – Cuts, sutures and costs: implementing policy and*
*monitoring standards – Patients and perseverance: grievances and resolution*
*– Sovereign remedies and preventive medicine: patient choice and markets –*
*Prognosis and preventive medicine: antidotes, tonics and learning –*
*Bibliography – Index.*

136 pp     0 335 09685 9 (Paperback)     0 335 09686 7 (Hardback)